Don't Weight

Eat Healthy and
Get Moving NOW!

Second Edition

Don't Weight

Eat Healthy and Get Moving NOW!

Second Edition

Kelly Bliss M.Ed.

Copyright © 2002 by Kelly Bliss, M.Ed.

ISBN 0-7414-0842-2

www.KellyBliss.com
www.buybooksontheweb.com
www.Borders.com
www.Amazon.com

Work it Out, Inc
Toll free 877-KellyBliss
(877-535-5925)

Published by:

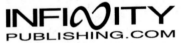

Infinity Publishing.com
519 West Lancaster Avenue
Haverford, PA 19041-1413
Info@buybooksontheweb.com
www.buybooksontheweb.com
Toll-free (877) BUY BOOK
Local Phone (610) 520-2500
Fax (610) 519-0261

Printed in the United States of America
Printed on Recycled Paper
Second Edition Published January, 2002

Dedication

This book is dedicated to
the disappearing ones.

May they find themselves
and take care of themselves.

Table of Contents

Acknowledgements

In the fall of 1980 I finished running my marathon, twenty-six miles and three hundred and eighty five yards. I only ran one. That was enough. In the winter of 1980 I was recovering from severe overuse injuries to my knees. I was also continuing my recovery from bulimia. As I think of these times, I realize I must first acknowledge the creative force that made my body and soul. I was given the awareness to hear what my body and soul had to teach me. I must express appreciation for the insight to understand the lessons that they were shouting. Somehow, back then, alone in the woods with my two little kids, I developed my own theory of self-acceptance and self-care. In the early 1980's I began teaching small classes using this wild new theory of healthy eating and fitness ... just because people deserve to feel good and be well ... not to lose weight. My body, soul, and awareness wrote the curriculum.

Fifteen years after my marathon, in 1995, I walked into the SCAN (The Sport, Cardiovascular and Wellness Nutritionists) conference in Baltimore Maryland. A dietitian named Dayle Hayes was speaking on a topic entitled "Feed Your Body, Move Your Body, Love Your Body". As she spoke, I was grateful that the auditorium was darkened. I sat there crying. I don't mean a tiny tear streaking down my cheek. I mean I was flat out sobbing. For the first time since I had thought up this wild idea of self-care and self-acceptance, I was not alone. I had colleagues. Dana Shuster and Dr. Alan King spoke on the treatment of diabetes with this self-accepting model. There were professionals in Medicine, Psychology, Education, Nutrition, Fitness and many others who believed that people have the right to self-acceptance and self-care independent of their weight. I had finally found the Size-Acceptance Movement. I was not alone and I wept for joy.

I want to thank all the people and organizations that have passionately fought for the rights of fat people. Two decades ago this battle was fought by The Fat Underground, Fat Chance, Fat Lip Readers, and a national organization called NAAFA (National Association to Advance Fat Acceptance). Now, professionals and lay people of all walks of life continue to make progress and make this small world a better place for large people.

Radiance Magazine and BBW (Big Beautiful Woman) Magazine have provided support for plus size living and have of given me the opportunity to reach thousands through my writing. These magazines have given large women a chance to see themselves as beautiful. They pave the way for self-acceptance and self-care in the heart of each woman who reads them.

All around the country there are events for people of size. Socializing, shopping, education, and activist events have changed the way the world feels to the people who have attended. I have often had the pleasure of speaking at these conferences and workshops. I give my thanks to each and every organization that has sponsored these life-affirming events. I give my thanks to the participants who have changed my life with their courage, honesty, and acceptance.

When I created my unique style of no-impact aerobics, it was because I had damaged my knees running a marathon. I learned how to provide fitness for people with knee injuries. Back then, I was a small person, so I learned how to design movement for small people. After my car accident and sleeping for most of two years, I became a bigger person. I continued my fitness and I learned how to design movement for bigger people. Yet, still, I did not really know how to design movements for very large people. I have Lynn McAfee to thank for that, and so much more. With her openness and body awareness, she taught me what a very large body needs to be safe when exercising. With her determination and courage she was willing to be my guinea pig as I designed movements for very large people who want to exercise. Since then I have had the pleasure of working with many very large people. I want to thank each and every one of them for the education they provided to me.

The foundation of my psychotherapy theory and practice is the problem solving process that I learned in Effectiveness Training that was developed by Dr. Tom Gordon and taught to me by Jean W. Dole M.A.

I would like to thank the Office of Vocational Rehabilitation for their help in continuing my business after my total disability with uncontrolled epilepsy. The Epilepsy Foundation of Southeastern Pennsylvania gave me vital support, education, and the opportunity to function as a role model for others who cope with the life altering condition of epilepsy.

I appreciate the many hours spent by my editors, Miriam Dole, Catherine Kelly, Joseph Patrick, Chris Polischuk, and Nicole M. Bliss. They have been so valuable in the writing of this book. Whatever errors you may find herein are mine and mine alone.

In closing, I would like to extend my heartfelt thanks to:

- My clients and class members who are my true teachers.
- My family, where I learned independence.
- My sister Catherine, who fought side by side with me in the diet and food wars for decades.
- My sister Mary, my first little girl, who taught me how good it feels to take care of the little ones.
- My daughter Nicole, who taught me about courage through her example.
- My son Adam, who I love now and forever.
- My Mother, who finally found peace with her weight and her body.
- My car accident and my epilepsy, because these were the worst things that ever happened to me, and the best things that ever happened to me.

Foreword

Part of a daily ritual for millions of people is weighing themselves. They feel "bad" or "good" depending on the number on the scale. Success is measured by those numbers. This is business as usual in a society that worships thinness. The irony is that, despite the cultural obsession with weight (and how to lose it), the average American is roughly 10 pounds heavier than his/her counterpart a generation ago.

The paradox is undeniable: We live in a weight-obsessed culture, with an estimated 50-70 million of us spending in excess of $30 billion annually in an effort to control our waistlines. Yet we're collectively heavier for the effort. Needless to say, "bad scale days" far outnumber the "good" ones. What are we to do?

Well, standard medical practice tells us to keep trying. Indeed the National Institutes of Health guidelines for treating men and women classified as either overweight or obese (based on the new body mass index), released in 1998, call for calorie restriction as the key component of treatment: cut calorie intake by 500-1000 calories per day for six months, in an effort to reduce body weight by 10 percent. To be sure, the guidelines also recommend physical activity. But the calorie-cutting approach to weight loss is clearly the main thrust. This is unfortunate. This approach has absolutely no chance of succeeding for all but a very, very tiny minority of "successful" dieters, and for millions may actually compromise the very thing that weight loss was supposed to improve--health.

This presents us with another paradox: Conventional wisdom tells us that obesity kills. Therefore, weight loss should improve the longevity prospects of obese people. The problem is that there is minimal scientific evidence to prove that weight loss will lengthen the lives of men and women medically classified as overweight or obese. To the contrary, some recent published evidence suggests that intentional weight loss may actually *increase* (yes, *increase!*) risk for premature death. Of course, the problem with such studies is so little is known about the subjects being studied…why they lost weight, how they lost weight, over what period of time, whether they maintained their weight loss, etc. And this raises another question about obesity as a "killer."

We have been told by the media that obesity is responsible for the premature deaths of some 300,000 Americans each year, second only to tobacco as a preventable cause of death in this country. This is a misstatement. The actual quote from the data synthesis in the New England Journal of Medicine Nov, 1993 is:

"The most prominent contributors to mortality in the United States in 1990 were tobacco (an estimated 400,000 deaths), diet and activity patterns (300,000)…"

The report did NOT say obesity caused these deaths. It said "POOR DIET AND PHYSICAL INACTIVITY" were prominent contributors to mortality. Therefore, I would like to comment on the activity levels of large people. For many reasons, large people tend to be less fit than their thinner counterparts. The physical characteristic of fitness is related to physical activity. Surveys also indicate that large people tend to be less physically active. It's likely that the higher death rates among large people observed in many epidemiological studies are due in part to low fitness levels, stemming from low levels of physical activity.

In fact, data from the ongoing Aerobics Center Longitudinal Study, conducted by researchers at the Cooper Institute for Aerobics, in Dallas, show that the apparent ill effects of body fat are completely negated by aerobic fitness.

*In other words, if you are physically active and fit,
body weight is irrelevant as
a predictor of life expectancy.*

Furthermore, data from the Cooper Institute reveal that "fat-fit" persons actually have much lower death rates that "thin-unfit" persons...proving that fitness is far more important than thinness in terms of health and longevity.

And this is why Kelly Bliss' new book, *Don't Weight: Eat Healthy and Get Moving Now*, is so important. As she makes abundantly clear, improved health and well being come about by making healthy choices in our daily living—the foods we eat and the activities we engage in—regardless of weight. The improved health and well being that accompany lifestyle changes are only minimally related to the weight loss itself, and mostly due to the direct effects of the lifestyle changes. Over the past 30 years or so, dozens of studies published in top-notch scientific and medical journals demonstrate unequivocally that health and fitness improvements accompanying lifestyle intervention are largely independent of changes in body weight or body fat.

So the choice seems obvious. We would be a whole lot better off, physically and emotionally, if we accepted the fact that healthy bodies can come in many sizes and shapes. Focus on things we can change, and accept the things we cannot. Kelly's book is an important contribution to the size-acceptance, non-diet movement.

Millions of Americans need to realize that the road to a fitter and healthier body is not so narrow as to prevent them from walking it.

Kelly's inspirational and reassuring book is a good traveling companion. To your good health and fitness, at any weight!

Glenn A. Gaesser, Ph.D.
Professor, Exercise Physiology, University of Virginia
Author of *Big Fat Lies: The Truth About Your Weight and Your Health*

About the Author

I see that many books include a section about the author in the back of the book. I introduce myself to you in the beginning of this book so that you will have a better sense of who is talking to you.

I am not a doctor or medical professional. I am a mental health professional, fitness specialist, and survivor of the weight loss wars. I have learned much from my struggles. Common sense if my greatest specialty. Problem solving is my most helpful skill.

I have been a practicing psychotherapist since 1987, with my Masters Degree in Psychoeducational Processes from Temple University. However, my real education and training as a psychotherapist did not come from the graduate school where I got my degree. I have been an ACE certified fitness professional and teacher of fitness professionals since 1980. However, the true source of my fitness expertise did not come from the workshops I attended and certifications I attained. Life taught me what I know. Over the decades, my clients have been my best teachers.

******

I was in grammar school in the 60's. I was the smallest kid in the class until puberty. At 13 I got some curves. I thought it was pretty cool. Mom and I went shopping for a dress to wear to the eighth grade trip. We found a nice hot pink suit. (This was the 60's after all.) We bought it one size too small. Mom said that it "would look great if I just lost five pounds". In order to get that hot pink suit to fit I did not eat for a week. It did fit, for one morning. As soon as I ate snacks on the bus, the skirt was too tight. I ended up wearing my jacket all day even though it was very hot. At 13 I knew I was too fat. At the time I wore a juniors size 9.

I was in high school in the 70's. I used to wear a 2" wide leather belt (that was pulled as tight as possible) to bed at night. I thought it would give me a better waistline. After all, wearing a ring made a dent in your finger. I thought a tight belt would do the same for my waistline. Of course, we all believed the lie that says: "a smaller waistline is better".

My mom always dieted. My sister was fat. I watched my sister be tormented by classmates, family members and doctors. I knew fat was bad. Eventually, I got blood blisters around my waist from the belt. I decided that big purple marks were as "ugly" as fat, so I stopped wearing the belt. I began a diet/binge cycle that was the gateway behavior to more serious problems.

In my twenties I taught "The Diet Workshop" for a major corporation and "Safe Slimming" at Pennsylvania State University Extension Service. I was compliant with the cultural norm of thinness.

At 19 I married my calculus professor. I was compliant with my husband's wishes. He wanted a house in the woods. I lived alone in the woods with my two small kids. He traveled all the time. I suffered and recovered from major depression, suicidal tendencies, and bulimia. The marriage was over in ten years. I got two smart kids and a great last name out of the deal. I decided not to be compliant anymore.

I used running as a crutch while I was letting go of my bulimia. I ran a marathon in 1980 with my sister. Time and time again, as my sister and I rounded a corner during the race, we heard: "Look, there are some fat ones!" That was the last straw. Right then and there I decided my body was naturally round. If running three hours a day had not made me thin, then nothing would.

The dieting was over forever. I would never over-exercise again. I would build a healthy lifestyle and trust that my body would be fine, at any size. I developed a therapeutic technique and life philosophy. I found motivation for my healthy lifestyle through pleasure and enjoyment, rather than through willpower and deprivation.

My thirties were a blast. I played hard. I worked hard. I became Unit Director of an urban mental health center. I learned so much from my clients. At age thirty-seven I was on my way to a meeting for the negotiations on opening a wellness center where I could combine mental health and fitness. On my way to a meeting, my car was rear ended while I sat at a stoplight. I suffered head trauma, developed uncontrolled epilepsy, and slept for most of two years while the doctors played with my medications. What an education! I learned more from my rehabilitation process than from graduate school.

With help from the Office of Vocational Rehabilitation, I started a business where I could provide self-accepting counseling and fitness even though my epilepsy remained uncontrolled. My daughter functioned as my "attendant" as I went through days in and out of seizures. Through phone counseling and video fitness, I began working with a variety of people including people with disabilities and very large people.

I developed such respect for the human spirit. I watched my clients solve their problems. I learned so much from the courage and creativity I saw in them every day. My clients have taught me hope. Hope is contagious.

In my private practice I often see people in excruciating pain: emotional, physical or both. The metaphor that comes to my mind at these times is an image of giving birth. In the midst of all this pain there is something wonderful being born. Often we don't know what it is. But there is always something emerging from the pain that is worth cherishing. All this pain ain't for nothing!

As you read this book, you will see lessons that I have learned from my courageous clients. You will see much of what I learned from my bulimia, suicidal depression, head injury, uncontrolled epilepsy, and my rehabilitation. These experiences were some of the labor pains for birthing a new attitude toward healthy living. This new attitude is what Don't Weight is all about. Enjoy.

Introduction

Do you want to feel better about your body? Do you want to build a healthy lifestyle? Good. These are goals you *CAN* achieve! These are goals that are constructive and self-esteem building. Self-nurturing goals like these are behind the growing *Self-Acceptance / Self-Care Movement* that has been building for over two decades. Self-acceptance helps people take better care of themselves. People who feel better about their bodies are more likely to succeed at maintaining healthy lifestyle changes than people who are self-critical and feel bad about themselves. According to Michael Kiernan, PhD, in a study done at Stanford University School of Medicine, "Members who started out more satisfied with their bodies, regardless of size, were more than twice as likely to succeed as their deeply dissatisfied counterparts (55% compared to 26%)."

In my psychotherapy practice, I see many people who are working on weight issues. Most of the people who are working on weight issues start out by wanting to lose weight as their primary goal. In my experience, at least half of those who want to lose weight have avoided social contact because they "felt too fat". Could it be that weight watching and the accompanying anxiety are contributing to social isolation? At least a third of my clients who started out watching their weight have reported staying at home and avoiding going out in public because they "don't want to be seen when they are this fat". Could it be that weight watching and society's negative attitudes toward fat are contributing to agoraphobia and other emotional problems?

The title of the book mentions healthy eating and fun fitness. Have you noticed what I have NOT encouraged? (You may have assumed that I was talking about it just because I promote healthy eating and exercise.) I have not encouraged weight loss or dieting. There is a very, very good reason for my omission.

Watching your weight is an ANXIETY, NOT an action ™.

In this book I propose we need new reasons to eat healthy and exercise. We need a new primary goal. I do not want to contribute to the negative effects, body loathing, and anxiety of watching your weight.

If weight loss were your primary goal, every action would be an exercise in self-criticism. If you were to focus on weight loss, you would be giving yourself the message that your body is wrong.

When healthy living is your goal, every action is an exercise in self-nurturing. When you focus on self-care and self-acceptance, your body is right where it should be ... with you on your journey toward wellness.

I encourage people to build a healthy lifestyle independent of weight. I recommend that you take action toward wellness, not weight loss. Specifically, I hope you will gradually let go of a focus on your weight and put your attention on your life. You deserve a good life. There are many aspects to making a good life. In this book I will primarily focus on motivation, eating, and fitness.

1.) In Chapter One we will look at the way you think about yourself, your body, your motivation, and the process of change.

2.) In Chapter Two we will explore a new way to make choices about food, emotional needs, and avoiding the "dieting vortex".

3.) In Chapter Three we will look at you, your body, and ways to stay fit in the body you have today.

4.) In Chapter Four we will pull it all together. We will look at "a day in the life" of Mary. A fictitious woman who demonstrates this new way of looking at self-care and self-acceptance.

As I received feedback on HOW people use this book, a pattern developed. This book is like an onion. It is likely that you will react and interact with it in layers. Often people sit down to read a section or two and find that they just keep reading all the way through. It is interesting. It is fun. It is like you and I sitting down and having a chat together. I AM talking directly to you. I have listened to people who cope with issues like yours. I have lived through many of the same things that you are living through right now.

Even if you read the book through, you may find it useful to go back and read it section by section. Like peeling back the layers of an onion, you will get closer to your central core issues regarding food, eating, body image, and your life. You will choose to revisit the sections that are most important to you. There are concepts to think about. There are psychological and awareness exercises to do. There are actions with which to experiment. This book is an EXPERIENCE. Give yourself time to have this experience over time. You will get more out of it if you try the actions suggested within your own life. Your awareness will grow more if you experience the new thought patterns for yourself as you live your day.

I often get the feedback that this book is like a warm island of acceptance and self-care encouragement. I suggest that you come back often and bathe in the warmth of these accepting attitudes.

You may find that you follow this pattern of reading the book and then going back to experience a section at a time. You may use this book in a completely different way. The choice is yours. Actually, that is the foundational premise of this process for healthy living:

The Choice Is Yours!
Tune in to what is going on INSIDE of you.
Increase your AWARENESS of what you need.
YOU CHOOSE the best way to meet your needs.
NOTICE if that way to meet your needs was effective.
If it was effective - ENJOY.
If it was not effective - make A NEW CHOICE.

This internally motivated process is the opposite of following a program that some external expert has formulated. With this internally motivated PROCESS you are always on your journey to self-care and self-acceptance!

Your body hungers for nutritious food. Your muscles ache for movement and exercise that feels good. Whatever your age, whatever your size, whatever your health status, whatever your abilities or disabilities, you CAN succeed at improving your wellness. You CAN eat healthy and start moving NOW!

For more information and support as you take your journey toward self-care and self-acceptance, check out **www.KellyBliss.com** When you sign up as a member (it is FREE to sign up) you will find:

1.) Your Online Workbook with exercises to help you understand yourself and make better choices.
2.) Your eNewsletter with motivation and information to help sustain positive motivation.
3.) Track Your Success to help you measure success without depending on the scale
4.) Much, much more!
Welcome to "Healthy Living with Bliss™"

Chapter One

A Fresh Way of Thinking

Guaranteed Success

Since you picked up this book, you are probably interested in healthy eating and fitness. You have probably worked toward these goals before. Perhaps in the past you ended up feeling like a failure when you did not follow through on your plans. Get ready for a new outlook on this old problem. With this fresh way of thinking, it is *impossible to fail* as you work toward your healthy lifestyle.

Yes, with this internally motivated process of self-care and self-acceptance you are guaranteed success! As long as you continue to participate in this process (which is very enjoyable and self-sustaining), you will continue to build your healthy lifestyle. Whatever you do (or don't do) when you look back on it, learn from it, *and make a better plan,* you are still on the path toward your goal. Throughout this book, I will use examples from the lives of my clients and from my life to demonstrate new ways to look at old problems.

The Trampoline

This is a true story. It happened in the early 1980's, but what Karla learned is timeless. She wanted to add some fitness to her life. It seemed impossible. She had so little time with her small kids and a huge house to tend. When she saw an advertisement for a "rebounder", a mini trampoline for exercise, she thought it looked fun. She thought that perhaps something fun would help her stop being so lazy. She got the trampoline and put it in the basement by the washer and dryer. She could workout anytime she was waiting for a load of wash to finish. As the weeks went by, Karla did not use her trampoline. She continued to call herself "lazy" in her own head. "This is such a small thing to ask of myself. What kind of lazy slob am I that I can't do this one simple thing?" This made her feel worse and worse. She felt like a failure.

One day, as she stood waiting for the wash, she asked herself a new question: "I wonder what stops me from using the trampoline?" The answer just popped out. "I can't jump on that thing without a good bra. All my bras are upstairs in my room, two floors up!" With a smile on her face, Karla ran upstairs, got several bras, and put them on hooks right by the trampoline. The next time she was waiting for a load of wash to finish, she conveniently grabbed a fitness bra off the hook on the basement wall. She didn't even take time to undress. She just put the bra right over her T-shirt and started jumping. Yep, she looked silly, but she was exercising! She kept exercising. She has been using the same type of problem solving ever since. She has been exercising, one way or another, for the last twenty years.

******

This story demonstrates how pushing with willpower is not enough. It shows how problem-solving and enjoyment are the real keys to success. In this book you will learn more about this problem solving process. You will learn more about finding motivation that is positive, constructive and self-perpetuating. It is impossible to fail at this process of building your healthy lifestyle. When you try to make a change in your lifestyle, either you make the change, or you don't. If you make the change (and if the change is comfortable enough to live with long term) you have a new habit. Fine, you have succeeded.

If you try to make a change and do not follow through, you have not failed. *You are just in the middle of the process.* Your next step is to look at the reasons your plans did not work out. It will take time to figure out what got in the way. It will take creativity to overcome the obstacles. It all starts with asking yourself "What got in the way?" When you answer this question and learn how to get over, around, or through the obstacles, you are closer to your goals. You have just taken the next step toward your healthy life. *You can take as many steps as you need.* You are in the process of building your healthy lifestyle. Fine, you are in the *middle* of succeeding. Since this process is *based on enjoyment and satisfaction*, you will want to continue. Therefore, you will succeed.

Process, Not Program

So, you want to eat healthy and get moving. You need to know what to do to accomplish this goal. There must be some program that will work for you. You have tried a hundred different food plans, diets, or nutritional programs. You have joined the gym or spa, paid your annual membership, then dropped out within a few weeks. What is going on? Where is the *program* that will finally work?

There is no program that will work. You will not find it at a seminar. It is not in a stack of audio-tapes. It is not even here in this book. There is no *program* that can tell you what to do to build your own healthy lifestyle. There is no external source for you to find what you need.

Don't worry, there is hope. *The hope is inside of you.* Learning to really listen to yourself and pay attention to what you need is the key. Yes, you can get good ideas from various programs. However, it is up to you to keep the ideas that are helpful and leave the ones that don't work for you. This is your own individual process, not a program.

Instead of following any one program, you will go through a process that is unique to you alone. In this book you will find tools, attitudes, motivations, behaviors, and skills to try out. You will also find encouragement for you to follow your own individual process.

How can you make use of all the wonderful information available on healthy living and not feel like you are participating in another "program"? *Change the WAY you look at the experts.* When you participate in a self-help group, take a fitness class, talk to a therapist, read a book on nutrition, watch a talk show, hear a news story, or see an infomercial, remember one fact: They may be experts in their fields, but there is only one real expert on the subject of you. That expert is YOU!

Teachers, instructors, counselors are *consultants that you hire* in order to get ideas and information. Books, talk shows, and seminars are places you look for information. You are in charge of trying out the new things that you have learned and deciding if they work for you. Every exercise, whether it is physical, emotional, or intellectual, is just an opportunity to experiment and see what effect it has on you. Tune in to yourself. How does it feel? Does it seem useful? Does it cause a problem? You decide. *You are the expert on you.*

There is nobody on earth who has the same needs as you do. There is nobody who knows you better than you know yourself. So, logically, you should be the one that you depend on as you go through the process of building your own healthy lifestyle.

In this book you will see some new ways of thinking about old problems. You can try out new behaviors. You can experiment with new motivations. This is a living, changing *process*, not just a program that you follow. Nobody else will travel exactly the same road that you will.

Most of the time, when people think of "eating plans", they think of a program that defines what to eat, portion size, when to eat, and other requirements of the program. By definition, a program has requirements and parameters that are set by some expert. Those who follow a program are supposed to learn the rules of the program and incorporate those rules into daily life. On any given day, you are either "on the program", or "off the program". You are either doing what the expert has told you to do, or you are not. When following a program, you always have a measuring stick available to tell how you are doing. The problem is, this measuring stick is usually used to criticize yourself and damage your self-esteem.

I do not offer a "program" for healthy eating and fun fitness. Instead, I offer a set of choices, tools, exercises, and insights. I propose or recommend new ways of looking at things and different actions to take. Each person will try these options in a different order and for a different length of time. Each person will select what works for them and what does not. No two people will choose the same path. This is your process for individual change. Your process will be unique. You have a very qualified expert to help you make the best choices ... that expert is you.

Keep an open mind as you choose your focus for each week. It is valuable to write down your goals. Writing goals is not a tool to force yourself to do something. It is a tool to increase your awareness of your ever-changing goals. You will not make a vow to achieve a specific goal no matter what. Instead you will keep adjusting your goals until they are just right for you and your life.

Sometimes you will do just as you planned. Sometimes you will not do as you had intended. That does not mean you failed. That means you have something to learn. IT IS AN

OPPORTUNITY TO FIGURE OUT WHAT YOU NEED. Was the goal more complicated than you had originally thought? Do you need to do something else *before* you can accomplish your original goal? If so, then you need to change your goal to reflect the new information.

I encourage you to select some action to take EACH WEEK that will affect your feelings, your fitness, and your healthy eating. Please only choose one small doable action or focus in each area. (If you try to do too many things, you will be overwhelmed.) When you write down your intentions at the beginning of each week, you will have something to reflect on at the end of each week. You will have the benefit of hindsight as you look back and compare your intentions with your real life. Did you do as you intended? What helped? What got in the way? Was there something you needed to do first, before you could accomplish your goal? How can you set yourself up to achieve your goals next week?

Keep thinking.
Continue to be creative and
try out new choices.
Set your goals and keep improving
on the goals that you set.

Listen to yourself.

You Can't Push a Rope

I would like you to picture a rope lying on the floor in front of you. If you wanted the rope to move, you could push it by one end. But you wouldn't do that. The rope would just bunch up in a tangled pile from that end. If you wanted to move the rope, you would PULL it. With very little effort you could move the entire rope with a single tug. When you think of motivating yourself to do anything, I want you to remember one thing: You can't PUSH a rope. You gotta PULL it!

Whatever is on your list of self-improvement, you will find more effective motivation when you PULL yourself towards your goals by noticing how *good it feels* when you accomplish your goal. When you eat something healthy, notice your sustained energy in the hours that follow. When you exercise, pay attention to the joy of moving your body. When you choose not to spend money, appreciate your reduced stress from lower credit card bills. Pull yourself toward your goals by increasing your awareness of what feels good about your new choices. This focuses on the benefit, not the task.

Too often we try to motivate ourselves with negative motivation. I hear people say: "When you get disgusted enough you will do something about it." This kind of thinking only encourages self-loathing. It eats away at your self-esteem. When you feel bad about yourself, you are least likely to have motivation to take care of yourself. Sometimes we try to motivate ourselves by thinking: "I should do this." or " I just need willpower to do this." When you try to push yourself to do things with "should" or "willpower", it is like pushing a rope. Pushing is exhausting. It focuses on the ***effort*** instead of on the ***benefit***.

- What do you want to motivate yourself to do?
- Do you want to feel better about your body?
- Do you want to improve your healthy eating?
- Do you want to include regular exercise in your daily life?
- Do you want better relationships with your friends and family?
- Do you want to manage your time or money better?
- Do you want to stop procrastinating?

What would PULL you toward your goals? Think about how *good it will feel* to take an action. Think of the *relief you get* when you complete a task. Think about the pleasure you will get from your accomplishment.

Feeling good IS great motivation.

When seeking motivation, focus on the enjoyment or benefit from accomplishing the steps that lead toward your goal. You will not be pushing with willpower.

**You will be pulling yourself
toward your goals with pleasure!**

Choose ACTION, not ANXIETY

You probably picked up this book because you wish you could include healthy eating and reasonable exercise in your life. Most people simply translate these behaviors into the concept of weight loss. In this book I do not make that assumption. When your lifestyle gets healthier, I do not know what will happen with your weight. I do know that you will be healthier and you will feel better about yourself and your body. These are positive outcomes independent of your weight.

**Watching your weight is an ANXIETY
NOT an action™.**

I encourage you to:
- Focus on self-care, independent of your weight.
- Choose the ACTIONS you can take toward self-care.
- Build a healthy lifestyle that meets your needs (both physical and emotional.)
- Learn problem-solving so that you can continually, and comfortably, adjust your lifestyle.

- Find motivation based on enjoyment and positive attitudes.
- Work toward self-acceptance and self-care.
- Pay attention to how you LIVE, not what you weigh!

To Weigh or Not to Weigh, That Is the Question

Let's look at how a focus on your weight would likely affect you:

At any given time of the year, an astonishing 15 to 35 percent of Americans are trying to lose weight. Think about a time when you were trying to lose weight. You may think about today, yesterday, or a decade ago. Remember getting on the scale (at a group meeting, a doctor's office, or in your own home.) Logically, there are three possible outcomes on the scale:

1.) You lose weight
2.) You gain weight
3.) Your weight stays the same

Of course, how you react to the scale depends very much on your eating before the weigh-in. Logically, there are three possibilities to describe your eating while trying to lose weight:

1.) You stuck to your eating plans
2.) You blew your eating plans
3.) Sometimes you stuck to your eating plans and sometimes you did not

Let's look at the likely reactions to weighing yourself, depending on how hard you worked on your eating plans.

Possibility #1. You stuck to your eating plans. First, we will look at the most frequent experience in the beginning of weight loss plans. After doing just as you planned for the week, you hopped up on the scale, and you lost weight. For the first week it probably was not that hard to do. You were psyched. You probably paid a lot of money for this plan. Even if you did not spend a penny, at the very least you had invested emotionally in this plan to lose weight. Now, after the first week, the scale told you that your weight was down. Good. All your efforts were worth it. You would stick to your eating plan. (But ... sometimes ... when the scale gave you good news ... didn't you just have to celebrate and eat something "illegal"? Oh, yeah, that will be talked about in possibility #2 and #3. Let's get back to possibility #1, sticking to your eating plans.)

Later on, however, the story changed. It became more and more difficult to have the willpower to stick to your eating plan. You did stick to it though. And, after all that effort, you needed a reward. You had worked too hard and you needed to see results on that scale. How would you feel if you saw that you had lost two pounds? Good. You probably would feel satisfied that your efforts were worth it. However, you and I both know that the human body does not react to caloric deprivation with sustained weight loss every week. The body adapts to the lower caloric input and eventually weight loss plateaus. It always does. Every time.

How would you feel when the scale told you that, after being so "good" and watching what you ate all week, you had lost only a half-pound, or stayed the same? What if, after all that effort, you had actually **gained** weight? It happens. It actually happens quite often.

If you did not get the results you wanted, what do you think weighing yourself would do to your motivation? Would you redouble your efforts, eating less and exercising more until the scale gave you the results you wanted? Many people do exactly that. This is not the most common reaction. But for the few who do take this path, this is often the beginning of an eating disorder. Or, would you react like most people do after working hard and getting no results? Most people lose their motivation and quickly or gradually stop working on losing weight. Unfortunately, since most people inexorably link healthy eating and exercise to weight loss plans, *most people also give up on their healthy lifestyle when they give up on weight loss.*

Possibility #2. You blew your eating plans. Next, we will look at another frequent scene as an approach is made to the scales. How many times have you been waiting in a line to be weighed and wondering if you "got away with it"? What if the scale "catches" you and reports that you did not lose any weight or even that you gained weight. How would that make you feel? Would this focus on the external measurement on the scale help you to tune into your inner self and figure out WHY you blew your eating plans? Would it help you understand yourself, your needs, or your life any better? Or, would this reprimand simply encourage you to "work harder"? However, if you worked harder, you would really need a reward when you got to the scale next time. What if, after working really hard next week, you gain weight when next you were weighed? (Oh, yeah, that is possibility #1. Let's get back to possibility #2.) So, in the next scenario, imagine that you ate a lot of foods low in nutrition, high in saturated fats and sugar. Still you lost weight. What would your reaction be to that? Would this positive report make you feel like it was fine to eat unhealthy foods? There were no negative consequences. After all, you did not gain weight. Could it be that this focus on your weight might take your focus OFF your nutrition?

Possibility #3. Sometimes you stuck to your eating plans and sometimes you did not. If you lost weight under these conditions, how would you feel? Would you feel like you "got away with it"? Perhaps you do not need to pay attention to your eating that much. Maybe next week you will "cheat" a little more and see if you get away with it. (Oh, yeah, that is possibility #2.) What if you stay the same or gain weight under these conditions? Would you need to get back on track and follow your food plan even more intently? Then, after all that effort, you would probably really need a reward from the scale when you get on it next time. (Oh, yeah, that is possibility #1.)

This is starting to sound so circular. Actually, most dieters report feeling trapped in exactly these destructive circular patterns or cycles. At times, when a dieter is temporarily in the "high" end of the cycle, things feel great. "My energy went right through the roof!" ...Temporarily. As the cycle continues, there is much pain, self-esteem bashing, feelings of failure, reduced awareness of the self, and the person becomes more and more distant from constructive motivations for healthy living. For the person who is working on an eating plan, there are negative psychological reactions lurking at every weigh-in. I have been working with people who want to lose weight for twenty-five years. I have NEVER known of anyone who had a consistently constructive reaction to the experience of getting weighed. Perhaps, there are better ways to measure the success of our efforts toward healthy living.

Yes, I recommend that you stop weighing yourself. For some of you, this will be a difficult process that requires much problem-solving and self-understanding. For others, you can just stop. Even when you go to the doctor's office, there is no reason why you should have to experience the negative effects of being weighed. If it is medically necessary to be weighed, just get on the scale BACKWARD and tell the nurse that you do not want to hear your weight. You may even choose to add that you are actively involved in a healthy living process, and it is detrimental to your process of healthy living to know your weight. If you don't know your weight, how will you know if you have succeeded?

Redefine Success

Let's face it, when people talk about improving their eating and fitness, they often measure success by getting on the scale. What is the reason for weighing yourself? Most of my clients say it is so they can tell if they have made any progress or so they will know if they have "succeeded". I suggest that you *measure your success in a different way*. In the beginning of each month ask yourself different questions and write down your observations:

- How is your breathing when you climb one flight of stairs, walk a block, or wheel your wheelchair around the mall?

Each person is in a unique situation when it comes to physical abilities and fitness. You cannot measure yourself against anyone else in order to get a clear picture of your success. Pay attention to your own physical capabilities right now. Whatever your abilities, appreciate them. Think about ways to gradually do a bit more physical activity than you did last month. As you take action and move a bit more you will be building your stamina. This is true whether you are a distance runner or a bed bound person doing your reclining aerobic workout. Every one of us is a corporeal being. We live in our bodies. When you use your body and cause yourself to breathe heavily, you are doing aerobics! When you do aerobic activity regularly, you will increase your aerobic capacity. That's GREAT! Notice your physical efforts. Appreciate your work. If you continue to do aerobic physical activity, you will be able to do more activity and breathe more comfortably than you did the month before. Your body will function better than it did the month before. Wow! That IS success!

- What is the intensity and duration of exercise that you are comfortable with at this time?

So, what *can* you do now? Whatever it is, you are at a great starting place. Notice the intensity at which you are able to work now. If you are a walker, notice how fast and how far you can walk. If you are a swimmer, notice what stroke and what pace is comfortable for you. If you use a wheel chair, how fast do you push as you travel on flat surfaces? How is your pace and control going up ramps?

When you notice the intensity of your workout, you will also be able to notice your improvement. After you have noticed the intensity of your workout, next be aware of how long you are participating in your activity of choice. You will be surprised at how your body responds to regular movement. You will be able to increase the duration of your exercise as you persist in staying active. It is important to appreciate the duration of your workout. However, you also need to write down your progress. It is too easy to forget how far you have come. Or, your high expectations could prevent you from appreciating your progress. By keeping a written record of intensity and duration of workouts, you will be able to SEE your progress and your success more tangibly.

- How are you sleeping? Are you able to fall asleep and stay asleep so that you wake up rested?

If you have no difficulty sleeping, this may seem like an overly simplistic measure of wellness. If you do have trouble sleeping, this may seem like an unattainable success. In either case, how you sleep affects how you feel. And conversely, how you feel affects how you sleep. When you exercise regularly, manage stress, and eat healthier, you will sleep better. Take the time to notice your sleep patterns. You may notice subtle improvements in how you feel that are worth appreciating.

- Notice your flexibility. Can you stretch a bit further than you did before you became more active? Do you feel less stiff?

Flexibility is one of the components of fitness and health that it is easy to ignore. Don't. Your flexibility if very important to your functioning. Including both strength and flexibility exercises in your routine will help to keep your body in balance and avoid injuries. Take time to notice your flexibility. This is another way to measure success where you have the power to affect the outcome.

- Are you eating more fruits and vegetables than you did previously?

Listen to the news. You will hear it everywhere. A diet that includes more fruits and vegetables is rich in phytonutrients--the natural vitamins and minerals from plants. Having more access to these complicated natural nutrients improves health and reduces your chances of getting many serious diseases. Put energy into figuring out HOW to include more tasty, enjoyable fruits and vegetables in your day. By the time you do all the problem-solving necessary to eat more "live" food, you will find you just naturally eat less of the foods that have little nutrition. I encourage people to pay attention to what they want to include in their food for the day, and never mind excluding any particular food. (We all know as soon as you tell yourself you will avoid or eat less of a particular food, THAT is just when you start craving it.)

- Are you choosing fats that are more heart healthy when you eat and cook?

Dietary fat, the fat in the foods you eat, is necessary for good health. How much fat should you include in your diet? What percentage is right for you? Experts have different opinions on this question. I suggest that you read what the experts have to say and then make a choice for yourself. I do not know how much fat you should eat. I DO know what KIND of fat you should choose as often as possible. There are volumes written on the subject, but I will boil it down to a few basic concepts:

1.) **Minimize saturated fat**. Saturated fat comes mainly from animal sources.
2.) **Minimize trans-fats.** Trans-fats act much like saturated fat in the body. When you see "partially hydrogenated fats" in the label, that means you will find trans-fats in the food.
3.) **Use monounsaturated fats more often** when you eat or cook with fat. These fats come from plants. Monounsaturated is best. (Oils like canola oil and olive oil have a high percentage of monounsaturated fat.)

If it makes you feel more comfortable, you can become much more of an expert on dietary fat. However, if you remember these basic concepts you can choose heart healthy fats in your eating and cooking.

Whenever you choose healthier fats, you are succeeding at taking care of yourself. If you want to notice your success, make some kind of record of the days when you have made better choices in this area. Some people like to write down elaborate records. Some people just put a "+" sign on the calendar on days when they have made better choices. I find that I respond well to stickers. When I am focusing on an area of my life that I would like to improve, like eating more heart healthy fats, I select a tiny sticker to represent my success. I get a real charge out of seeing all those stickers pile up on my calendar. I don't have to rely on the scale to see my success. Success is staring at me in blazing colors on my calendar!

• Are you drinking more of the water your body needs?

This is not as simple as it sounds. Later in this book we will look at HOW to get more water into your day. For now, I would like to point out two things. First, as we all know, water is good for you. Second, as most of us have experienced, many diets include drinking lots of water as a diet strategy. Please, please, don't use drinking water as a way to lose weight. That is the surest way to begin to HATE drinking water. That will probably result in you drinking less water and not feeling as well as you could. I have seen clients reduce headaches, improve energy, and minimize swelling, just by hydrating their bodies properly. I encourage you to drink more water just because your body deserves to feel better, not to lose weight. When you succeed at drinking more water, you have succeeded at improving the health of your lifestyle. Good. Appreciate your success.

- What is your resting heart rate? One morning upon awakening, before you even get up, just lie there and take your pulse. That is your resting heart rate. Is it any lower than it used to be?

Your resting heart rate is a good monitor for your fitness. It does not matter what it is when you start out. Don't fret about what your resting heart rate is when you first take it. All that matters is that, with regular aerobic movement, you *can* lower your resting heart rate as time goes by. This will be a gradual process. Every little bit counts. As you increase the efficiency of your cardiovascular system through regular exercise, your heart beats slower. That is great for your health in many ways. When your resting heart rate is slower, that means you are more fit. That is a great measure of your success.

- How are your cholesterol and blood pressure?

Again, it does not matter what your cholesterol and blood pressure are when you start out. There is no value in judging yourself for where you are now. Life is complicated. The human body is more complicated. Your physical condition is a dynamic process. Right now, you can have a positive effect on that process by making better health choices starting today. Please do not judge your current cholesterol and blood pressure measurements. It does not matter where these measurements are when you start. It does matter that they improve gradually over time and stabilize at a healthy level for you. When you notice and keep track of the improvements in these measurements, you will have another real measure of success.

- If you have a medical condition like diabetes, glaucoma, arthritis, fibromyalgia, chronic fatigue, or one of the many other conditions that improve with fitness, notice the current status of your condition in the beginning of each month. Is there any improvement since last month?

When coping with chronic illness sometimes you feel dramatically better or worse. Big changes are easy to notice. However, more often you experience subtle changes in the way you feel. These subtle changes are easy to miss if you do not have a system for noticing them. When you write down how you are feeling, you will increase your awareness of the changes in your medical condition. Frequently I see clients who have been improving so consistently and so gradually that they did not even notice the difference until we noticed it together in a session. Likewise, people sometimes feel worse so gradually that they don't really notice the downward spiral. This can result in missing the opportunity to take corrective action sooner rather than later.

Regular appropriate fitness has a beneficial effect on many chronic illnesses. Eating more nutritious foods gives your body the building blocks necessary to heal and cope with physical problems. Notice how you are feeling. Keep a written record of your progress. If there are specific measurements that reflect the status of your chronic illness, find out what those measurements are and keep track of them. You will feel more empowered when you see the effect your lifestyle has on your physical condition. You will become a person who manages your illness instead of being the victim of it. That is success!

- How are your relationships? Have you enjoyed contact with supportive people? Have you reduced contact with hurtful people?

These are very important questions. Human beings do not live in a vacuum. People are affected by each other. Whether you live alone or you are in a large bustling household, people affect you. Pay attention to how you react to the people in your life. When you are around some people you may feel comfortable, accepted, and valued. When you are around other people you may feel criticized, judged, and like you can't do anything right. When you notice how people affect you, you can make better choices.

You can improve your relationships by taking specific steps to do so. Improving your communication skills and practicing better relationship skills can help. Read, take classes, join support groups, and/or get therapy. Make yourself the best partner you can be when you participate in your relationships. You can also manage your exposure to people who affect you in different ways. You may choose to spend more time around supportive people. You may choose to limit your time around hurtful people.

Sometimes you will find the same person is both supportive at times and hurtful at times. There are many ways to cope with this situation. I would like to describe one simple way: If someone is hurtful when they talk with you on a specific topic (like weight, dieting, body loathing comments, etc.), then set boundaries with that person and tell them that you don't want to discuss these specific topics with them. You may find that you have to resist your own tendency to bring up the very same topics with this person. It can help to have another topic ready to go in order to encourage both of you to avoid the topics that are hurtful within this relationship. Try it. You may find that you have many other constructive things to talk about. (Note: You may talk about the same topics with someone else and feel very supported and accepted. It is not the topic itself that may be hurtful. It is the topic within a relationship that includes judgment and criticism.)

You do not have to participate in or endure hurtful relationships. You do have the right and responsibility to enjoy constructive relationships. When you build better relationships, you will get the support you need to take better care of yourself.

- How are your stress levels? Have you taken small steps toward having more effect on your environment, your schedule, your workload, etc?

Stress is not necessarily bad. Some stress is what makes life exciting and interesting. The problem comes when there is too much stress and when the stress is continuous. The human body responds to stress by engaging the "fight or flight" systems. Many physiological changes take place in order to prepare the body for combat or escape. Our blood vessels constrict, blood pressure rises, heart rate increases, the hormone cortisol (among others) is released, and alertness and anxiety heighten. Back in the day of the cave man, these responses happened quickly, and then subsided quickly when the stress went away. In modern times, the stress is often continuous. We are often left with the emotional and physiological effects of stress affecting our bodies and our health continuously for days and weeks and years on end.

Stress makes any ailment or illness you have worse. Stress prevents you from healing as fast as you could. Stress increases depression and anxiety. Yeah, yeah, you know that. But what can you do to REDUCE STRESS? The answer may surprise you.

**Figure out ways to have an effect
on what happens in your life.**

It sounds so simple. It really works. You do not need to control your life. You just need the power to make small doable changes in your life. You will feel less stress when you feel yourself having an effect on your environment, schedule, workload, etc.

You can be the person managing your problems,
instead of the victim of them.
This reduces stress.

Stress is the feeling you get when your problems run you over like a Mack truck. You can reduce your stress by climbing up into the driver's seat and having an effect on the path that the truck takes. You still have problems, but now you can DO something about them! You have an effect on your life.

Each month take time to notice your stress levels. Appreciate the small steps you have taken to affect your life. Write down how you feel and what helped you to feel better. These are subtle things. If you do not take time to notice and record them, you might miss an opportunity to savor part of your success. You deserve to see progress when you work on your healthy lifestyle.

Measure your success by your actions, your increasing abilities, and how you feel. You can add your own questions that will help you measure success! Here is the above list of questions in consolidated form:

- How is your breathing when you climb one flight of stairs, walk a block, or wheel your wheelchair around the mall?
- What is the intensity and duration of exercise that you are comfortable with at this time?
- How are you sleeping? Are you able to fall asleep and stay asleep so that you wake up rested?
- Notice your flexibility. Can you stretch a bit further than you did before you became more active? Do you feel less stiff?

- Are you eating more fruits and vegetables than you did previously?
- Are you choosing fats that are more heart-healthy when you eat and cook?
- Are you drinking more of the water your body needs?
- What is your resting heart rate? One morning upon awakening, before you even get up, just lie there and take your pulse. That is your resting heart rate. Is it any lower than it used to be?
- How are your cholesterol and blood pressure?
- If you have a medical condition like diabetes, glaucoma, arthritis, fibromyalgia, chronic fatigue, or one of the many other conditions that improve with fitness, notice the current status of your condition. Is there any improvement since last month?
- How are your relationships? Have you enjoyed contact with supportive people? Have you reduced contact with hurtful people?
- How is your stress level? Have you taken small steps toward having more effect on your environment, your schedule, your workload, etc?

It is useful to write down your responses to these questions about once a month or so. Keep your written answers in your own book. This will help you to see your progress over time. You will find motivation to continue your healthy lifestyle when you give yourself a concrete record of your improvements.

**Measure your success by noticing
the changes and improvements in**
- **how you feel**
- **what you can do**
- **your health status**
- **your life**

Measure your success by the improvements in your wellness, happiness, and lifestyle. *These improvements will keep you motivated more effectively than a scale ever could.*

"Your Own Book"

When I was commenting on ways to measure your success without paying attention to your weight, I mentioned that you might write down your progress and keep your writings in "Your Own Book". This is a tool for developing awareness of what you need, how food affects you, how you react to activity, etc. For now, I call it "Your Own Book". Get a blank book or a notebook that feels good to you. (You can also order the Healthy Living with Bliss™ Journal to record your journey. Or you can order the Don't Weight™ Workbook with exercises, experiences, and questions already included. Check out **www.KellyBliss.com** or call toll free **1-877-KellyBliss** to order the right one for you.)

Select a time in your day when you will regularly write in "Your Own Book". You decide if it is morning, noon, or night. Find a place where you can sit down and tune in. Throughout this book (Don't Weight) you will find several suggestions for possibilities of what you might write and what questions you may choose to answer for yourself. It is up to you to choose the sequence and content of Your Own Book. You may choose to ignore some questions or topics. You may put the last one first and the first one in the middle. You may write on one topic each day or you may stay on one topic for weeks. You're the expert. Do what you choose.

It is up to you to give "Your Own Book" a title. How do you know what title you want to give it until you know what you will discover as you write it? I do have a suggestion for a temporary title to use for now until you discover your own title: *I Wonder What Title I Will Discover for My Own Book.*

When you write, you do not need to worry about spelling or sentence structure. Many people prefer to use bulleted lists instead of sentences. You choose the format that suits you. You're the expert. If you do not like to use writing as a tool, you could choose to think, or draw, or sing about the ideas and questions that come up. Even if you choose not to write, you might try working on these issues at the same time each day in order to give some structure to your process. In that case you could keep your mind open to discover the "title" for your unfolding train of thoughts, or pictures, or songs. I will use the phrase "write your own book" to include your writing, thinking, drawing, or singing, whichever works for you.

I Wonder

We all talk to ourselves in our heads and out loud. The way you talk to yourself is very important. Every time you repeat a negative thought, you make it more likely to be true. For example, The more often you repeat, "I can't think of a title for my book", the more likely it will be that you will not be able to think of a title. When you change the way you talk to yourself and say, "I wonder what title I will discover for my book", you have left your mind open for the positive to surface and be recognized. Using phrasing that starts with "I wonder" is an important skill.

- Instead of: "I can't do that", try saying: **"I wonder what will help me to do that."**
- Instead of: "I don't know what I really want in life", try saying: **"I wonder what I really want in life"**
- Instead of: "I can't tell how I feel", try saying: **"I wonder how I feel"**
- Instead of: "I never finish anything", try saying: **"I wonder what will help me finish this"**

Wondering is wonderful! "I wonder" leaves your mind open to ideas that may help solve the problem. As you write in "Your Own Book" you will have plenty of opportunities to practice this powerful rephrasing. Does this sound like a useful exercise to you? If it does, you may choose to write about your experience with this exercise in "Your Own Book". Think about the way you think.

As you become aware of how often you talk to yourself in negative ways, you may be surprised at how frequently you do it. You may begin to feel bad for being so negative so often. Remember, you were taught to use these negative phrases. And, you can LEARN to use more helpful phrases. I encourage you to notice your negative thinking ... and be happy every time you are aware of a negative thought or phrase. Every time you notice a negative thought, YOU HAVE THE OPPORTUNITY TO CHANGE THE WAY YOU THINK. Your increased awareness is the key to changing and improving your life. This opportunity for improvement is part of your road to success.

Flipping the Coin: Finding the Positive

Every time you think a critical thought, say hurtful things to yourself, or participate in negative self-talk, you are damaging your self-esteem. You see, **you believe what you hear,** especially from yourself. This kind of negative thinking or self-talk is like a burrowing insect that eats away at your self-esteem and self-confidence. You do not have to be the victim of this hurtful process. You can turn it around and brush away that burrowing insect of self-criticism.

The first step to reducing hurtful and negative thoughts is to increase your awareness of when you are saying hurtful and negative things to yourself. Listen to the way you talk to yourself. Would you say those same things to another person? Would you talk like that to someone who was entrusted to your care? Would you speak that way if you wanted to encourage somebody?

**If a thought or comment would be hurtful
when addressed to someone else,**

**then it would be hurtful
when thought or said to you.**

You may find that you even criticize yourself for even having negative thoughts. Don't. You have a better option. When you notice that you just talked to yourself in a negative way, don't feel bad that you "did it again". Instead, feel good that you intercepted that negative thought. Feel good that *you are increasing your awareness!* You must first notice that you participated in negative self-talk before you can begin to stop it. The question is; what do you DO when you notice negative self-talk? The answer: DISAGREE. Disagree thoroughly. Disagree vehemently.

Think or say your disagreement in your mind with full sentences, in full paragraphs, with expletives. Or you can speak out loud about your disagreement (this works best if you are alone somewhere.) The more clearly you voice your disagreement, the more you can brush away the burrowing insect of self-criticism. It really works. Your clear positive statements to yourself prevent you from believing the old negative thoughts that you were taught.

Cloe

At forty-seven years old, Cloe was thinking about going to college. These were the thoughts running through Cloe's mind as she was trying to make the decision:

(Negative thoughts)
- College is for kids and I'm too old.
- I've been uneducated for this long, what's the difference if I spend twenty more years uneducated?
- I can't do this. I'm not smart enough. I'm not good enough.
- There is no reason for me to go back to school.
- I can never make decisions. I don't even know what I want to do with my life.

If Cloe had a friend who was thinking about going to school, would she say those kinds of things to her friend? I don't think so. If Cloe's adult son were making this same decision, would she speak to him this way? I don't think so. Suddenly, Cloe had realized she was saying nasty things to herself that she would never say to other people. With that realization, she had the opportunity to change. She could stop her negative self-talk by disagreeing vehemently with those old hurtful concepts she had been taught. She found herself saying instead:

(Positive thoughts)
- Anybody can go to college. I have every right to go to college! I like using my mind. I enjoy learning.
- I have learned a lot from the education life has given me so far. Now I want to add some formal education to the knowledge I have already acquired.
- I can do this. Of course I'm smart enough. I am a valuable person. I am a good person.
- I have many reasons to go back to school. I have practical, financial, and emotional reasons to go back to school. My reasons count. My reasons matter.
- I have the courage to struggle with making decisions, even though it is difficult for me. I will think it through. I will use my courage to persevere and make a choice. I have made a million choices in my life. I WILL make this choice too.
- Life is such a wonder. Here I am at forty-seven and the doors are wide open. My life is an unwritten book and I am the author. I can write what I want on those pages. How exciting. I get to decide what I want to do with my life. MY life.

******

Yes, Cloe did vehemently disagree with the first list of negative thoughts. She disagreed at length, in full sentences, in full paragraphs. Can you imagine that those negative thoughts would be pretty far away by the time she thought about these positive topics for a while? She did not let the burrowing insect of self-doubt get in and eat away at her self-esteem. It worked.

At fifty years old she had completed her associates degree. Now, at the time of this writing, she has completed her Bachelor's Degree! She is still open for what she wants to do with her life. She is excited! There is great power to being able to "flip the coin" and turn negative into positive.

You can actually construct the positive image of yourself in your mind by disagreeing with the negative. You can flip the coin and experience yourself as a more positive person. You too can literally rebuild your self-esteem, just like Cloe!

A Ghost In Your Closet

There may be someone else in your house who has the power to damage your self-esteem. They often lurk in your closet or in a basement storage area. This ghost may be about the same size you used to be. This ghost may be the size you wish you were. You can be plunged into bad feelings just by thinking about this ghost that haunts your closets. Are you saving clothes that you used to wear (or clothes you bought and never could wear), just in case this ghost shows up again? Who is it? It is you. It is the person you used to be when you were thinner and younger, or the person you wish you were when you bought that outfit one size too small. It is the "ghost of sizes past".

> **Every time you wish for the**
> **"ghost of sizes past" to return,**
> **you are criticizing and rejecting**
> **the person who you are right now.**

Waiting for this ghost hurts you.

**That self-criticism can eat away
at your self-esteem.**

In the long run, that self-criticism can also drain away your motivation to take better care of yourself. How many years can you stare at a closet full of clothes that do not fit before you become hopeless that they will ever fit? When you are hopeless, what is the use? "I'll never get back into those clothes, I might as well give up." What is it that you give up on? Usually, you give up on eating healthy and exercising.

**The ghost in your closet can CAUSE you
to give up on your healthy lifestyle!**

Go to your closet and open it. Do you see things in there that you cannot wear because they no longer fit you? How does that make you feel? Remember that feeling bad about yourself sucks away your motivation to take care of yourself. Are you saving these clothes in case you get back to that size again? Even if your body size changed and you end up the same size as these clothes from the past, the styles would have also changed. You would have changed. You are not and will never be the person you were in the past. This is a good thing. Think of all that you have learned, all that you have been through. You *should* look different than you used to look. Time moves forward. Get rid of the ghosts hiding in your closets that make you feel bad about yourself. You could donate those clothes to charity, give them to a favorite niece, or sell them at a resale shop. These clothes can make someone else feel good. Get rid of clothes that don't fit. It will make you feel better about yourself when you open up your own closet.

On the other hand, when you look in your closet, do you see clothes that *do* fit you? Do you find the clothes you need to get through your days comfortably? If not, what are you waiting for?

I would like you to imagine that you were in charge of caring for a child. Now, think of this little one who is in your care and notice how you would treat this child. Would you force that little one to wear clothes that do not fit? Would you deny him/her comfortable clothes that look nice?

If you were dressing a little one in your care, you would make sure that little one was dressed appropriately ... even if the little one were going to change body size soon! You would not force a three year old to go without clothes just because he/she will need a different size next year.

Even if you expect your body size to change, you deserve to have clothes that fit NOW.

If you give yourself any less, you are subjecting yourself to the same kind of judgment and neglect that would hurt anyone. Perhaps, when you were a child, you were hurt in this same way. Don't continue the damaging pattern.

Go ahead. Get rid of the ghosts in your closet and fill your closet with acceptance.

This does not have to cost a lot of money. If you cannot buy clothes right now, just move the things that don't fit into boxes somewhere out of sight and put the things that do fit closer to the front of the closet and drawers. If you have a little money, there are stores with budget prices, resale shops, and clothing swaps. Of course, if your finances allow, it is wonderful to treat yourself to something extra nice. You will find a resource for plus size clothes for men, women, and children at www.PlusSizeYellowPages.com

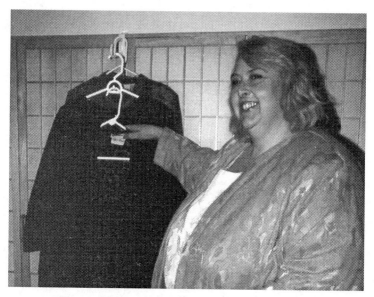

People of all sizes, even very large size people, can shop for clothes that fit. For hundreds sellers of plus size clothes of ALL sizes see www.PlusSizeYellowPages.com

Having clothes that fit is an *experience* of self-acceptance. Your experiences affect how you feel. People often ask me "HOW do I learn to accept my body?" There are many answers. There are many paths to self-acceptance. It always helps to take an ACTION toward your goals. Set up your closets and drawers so they are filled with clothes that fit your body NOW. This is one action you can take toward self-acceptance and feeling better about your body. Feeling better about yourself helps keep you motivated to take care of yourself.

A Gift to Myself
(One of My True Stories)

A question used to rule my life. I didn't realize it until one holiday season. There was a question in my head that was draining the fun out of my holidays. I mention holidays, because that is when I had this experience. You can think of any extra-stressful time in your life: preparation for a wedding, family visits, religious events, etc.

When I awakened each day I would ask myself, "What do I *have* to do today?" I asked this all the time, but especially during the holidays when there was so much to do. I thought this question would help prioritize my jobs for the day. I didn't realize it was causing a problem. It seemed to be a simple enough question. It was just the wrong question.

When I thought about what I *had* to do, I focused on the tasks in front of me. During the holidays, that was overwhelming. In addition to the usual family, home, and business responsibilities, I had all the holiday preparation too. By the time I added shopping, decorating, and cooking to the list of jobs, I didn't even know where to start. Frankly, it was depressing. This overwhelming list of jobs was sucking the fun right out of the holidays. I needed a new question:

"What do I want to give myself today?"
Instead of focusing on the list of jobs I had to do,
this question focused on the
reward for doing a single job.

Think about this question in your own life. Choose what reward you want, and give it to yourself. This works with housework, holiday tasks, and family responsibilities. If the kitchen is a mess, instead of thinking that you *have* to clean it up, think about how nice it will be to have a warm holiday drink sitting in your beautiful kitchen. Give yourself the gift of a nice clear counter and table. Instead of dreading the job of wrapping presents, give yourself the gift of relief from stress. You deserve that sense of relief you will feel when the presents are wrapped and sitting in a pretty pile. Give yourself that sense of relief sooner rather than later.

Think of your "to do" lists. These lists contain all the things you need to do. Sometimes these lists can be useful. More often they make you feel overwhelmed. From now on I encourage you make "to give" lists instead. On your "to give" list you note what you want to give yourself, and the tasks that are involved. This new list will help you focus on the reward or benefit from doing each task, instead of on the task itself. This list can increase self-knowledge and your awareness of your motivation. It is less overwhelming. Here are some examples:

I want to *give* myself *relief from stress* by:
- paying bills
- gathering tax information
- finishing a task

I want to *give* myself the *sense of accomplishment* from:
- finishing my resume
- cooking a nice dinner
- fixing the broken table

I want to *give* myself *nurturing* by:
- packing a healthy lunch
- moving my body with swimming
- saying "No" when I am overextended

You deserve to focus on the enjoyment and benefit from your accomplishments. Instead of asking yourself what you *have* to do, ask yourself **"What do I want to give myself?"** This new question has changed my life. It can change yours too.

Back Up, Don't Beat Up

What about the times when you really CAN'T get yourself to do something? You have tried and tried and you just don't do it. What then? It is very normal to beat yourself up. Most people have *learned* to reprimand and berate themselves when they "fail". You can develop a new way to think about things and replace the old unhelpful way of thinking.

**When you try to get yourself to "just do it",
and you "just don't do it",
there is always an obstacle.**

**There is ALWAYS a reason.
It could be an internal or an external reason.**

**Instead of beating yourself up,
think about the obstacle that might be in the way!**

Figure out a way around it, through it, or over it. Continue to problem solve and figure out what the obstacle is and how to cope with it. You are not a failure. You are on the path to accomplishing your goal. You are just in the middle of figuring it out.

Ask yourself what is getting in the way of accomplishing your goal: "I wonder what the obstacle might be." Open your mind and feelings to discover the possibilities. Keep your mind open and wonder about what those obstacles might be for as long as it takes. You do not have to come up with an idea right away. It may take days or weeks of wondering before you discover what the real obstacle might be. Once you know what gets in the way, you can make plans to solve that problem. When the obstacles are removed, when the problems are solved, you will easily be able to move forward. The best place to look for what gets in the way of accomplishing your goal is *behind* you.

Good Morning

Mike had plans. He was going to get up every morning and work out. He planned to begin by using a video workout right in his own home for convenience. He started out great. He got up every morning for a week and a half. Once in a while, when he was too tired, he skipped a workout. He told himself that he would get right back on track tomorrow. Then, inexplicably, he just was not doing his workout. He did not know what had changed. He just could not make himself get out of bed to do it.

At first he berated himself and called himself names. "What the hell is the matter with me that I can't do this one thing?" It did not take long for Mike to notice this train of thought was not fixing anything. As a matter of fact, the more he beat himself up, the more he felt like a failure. The worse he felt about himself, the harder it was to find any motivation. He had to approach this in a different way.

"I wonder what is getting in the way of my morning workouts?" A groggy answer slowly formed in Mike's head: "I'm too tired." Now, Mike had something to work with. But that was only the beginning. At first he thought that all he had to do was go to bed earlier. He tried for days to get to bed earlier, but he couldn't. O.K., Mike had to ask himself: "What is getting in the way of my early bedtime?" He was doing office work in the evening. How could he possibly get his work done at the office so that he did not have to bring work home? Mike ended up restructuring his entire workday, getting to bed a little earlier, and resumed his morning workout. He had to back up, and keep backing up, solving one problem at a time, in order to give himself the good morning that he deserved!

******

Think about your own life and your goals. Let's say you wish that you were eating healthier foods. You look at your day, and you decide that you have a rather simple plan for healthy breakfasts. A few days go by and you do indeed succeed with your breakfast plans. You are taking this self-improvement one small step at a time so you can continue to feel successful. Good.

Now, you are ready to work toward healthy lunches. You intend to pack a lunch and bring it to work. That seems simple. It should be easy enough. You will just make yourself do it. Well, time went by, and you just did NOT do it. You don't know why. You may think to yourself: "It was such a simple thing. Anybody can pack a lunch. What the heck is wrong with me that I could not accomplish this one little thing?"

If you ever experienced this kind of thinking, you were "beating yourself up". It is normal to beat yourself up. It is just not helpful. Let's look at this thought process and see where you can change your way of thinking. Let's see where you could learn to "back up, don't beat up".

The choice to eat healthier lunches makes sense. It is the next thought, the idea "it is such a simple thing", that is just plain incorrect. Packing your lunch and getting ready to pack your lunch is not simple. It is the end result of a complicated process. In order to pack your lunch you have to "back up" and do some problem solving. Think about the morning to see if you have allowed enough time to pack lunch. If you need more time in the morning, you may need to back up and change your evening routine so that you can get up earlier.

Upon reflection, you may decide to pack your lunch the night before. What do you need to change about your evening routine in order to accomplish this? Do you have the ingredients for a healthy lunch? Do you need to incorporate a shopping trip into your week to make sure you have what you need? Back up again. What changes will you need to make to fit the shopping into your life? It goes on and on until you have solved the problems that got in the way of accomplishing your goal.

Did you notice? This is NOT simple! It is very achievable, but it is not simple. It is challenging. If you had known that this was a challenging task, then you would have been more patient with yourself, more likely to problem-solve, and more likely to accomplish your goal. You would have been more prepared to "back up". *When you acknowledge that you are engaged in a challenging task, you increase your chance of success.* Any goal that you do not achieve on the first attempt is a good opportunity to practice the skill: "back up, don't beat up".

Motivation is Like a Big Balloon

I don't know why, but for me, I think of a big red balloon. As you hear what I have to say, you will have to decide what color your balloon will be.

Picture your balloon. Imagine you have drawn your face on it. Whenever you think a positive thought about yourself, or ask a positive question, your balloon inflates. Whoosh! You can practically hear the air whoosh in. Whenever you deride yourself or say something negative to yourself, your balloon deflates. Eeee! The air seeps out with an ominous squeak.

This is a great metaphor for your motivation. When you feel bad about yourself, things seem hopeless and out of your reach: "What a slob", "Why can't I do this one simple thing", "I'm just lazy", "I never finish anything". I hear it. Do you? Eeee! Your motivation is seeping away. Your balloon is deflated and immobilized. You feel unable to succeed.

Fortunately, the opposite is also true. When you feel good about yourself, things seem possible. You feel your ability to affect your life and your situation: "That sure was a good start", "I wonder what clever solution I will find?", "I'm in this predicament for some reason, I wonder what I will learn?", "I sure gave myself a good morning", "That felt great". Whoosh! Your motivation is whooshing in. Your balloon is big and bright. You feel able to succeed.

Pay attention to how you talk to yourself. Notice how you think about yourself. Once you are aware of hurtful messages you give yourself, you can change your mind and give yourself constructive messages.

You may want to use writing on this topic to solidify this concept for yourself. What color is your balloon? Do you want to increase your awareness of what positive things you say to yourself? Would you like to increase your positive statements? Think about it and write some down that would apply to today. Are you a visual person? You might want to include some drawing or graphic of your balloon in your writing. When I wrote in "My Own Book", I actually put a balloon in an envelope taped to the page. That way I could actually take it out and blow it up. Feeling the air go in, hearing the air squeak out, really helped me to keep the concept in my head. Experiment with yourself and find what works best for you.

Think of your balloon and remember that positive thoughts will keep you motivated. Cultivate your positive thoughts. Practice appreciating your accomplishments *and* your efforts. Notice what makes you feel bad and reduce your exposure to those people, places, things, thoughts, and experiences. Motivation is not an accident or a serendipitous event. Motivation is cultivated by *actively* practicing the skill of positive (non-critical) thinking.

Ride the Wave

Clients often come to me seeking control of their eating, control of their body size, control of their lives. This is a metaphor to express a new outlook on control.

Think of a lake, a big lake. This is a fresh water lake that is large enough to freeze at times or to have big waves at times. (Can you tell I grew up along Lake Michigan?) Imagine that the water is your life. Your job, as you live your life, is to stay on top and not sink. You could put all your energy into maintaining a great big condenser and freeze the lake solid in the area around you. It would take continuous energy to keep the water frozen. Then you could stay on top by walking on the solid surface in the small area around yourself. You would feel like you were in control. You would have to put all of your energy into maintaining that control. You would have to stay focused on the one small area that you have managed to keep frozen. You would be in control as long as nothing else happened to take your energy or focus away from maintaining that frozen patch.

Doesn't that sound a lot like staying on a diet, maintaining obsessive-compulsive tendencies, or participating in eating-disordered behavior? You can keep it up until something in life happens that takes your energy and focus elsewhere. When I worked for weight loss companies, I used to teach people how to cultivate obsessive or compulsive behaviors that would keep all their energy focused on controlling food. Indeed, when I read stories or see news reports of individuals who belong to the Weight Loss Registry (a national database at The University of Pittsburgh Medical Center that contains information on 3000 people who have lost weight and kept it off for at least a year), I see lots of obsessive or compulsive behaviors. One man proudly displayed stacks of notebooks where he had written down *every bite of food he had eaten for the last twenty years.* Another woman talked about her THREE hours of exercise daily to control her weight.

If someone who weighed ninety-eight pounds performed these very same behaviors, they would be considered eating-disordered behaviors. Why should these extreme behaviors be encouraged just because someone weighs one hundred and ninety-eight pounds?

I do not recommend odd behaviors like this. I do not recommend controlling your weight. That would be too much like trying to maintain the frozen patch on the lake. Instead, I suggest you learn new skills that will keep you safe, even though the water is fluid and ever changing. I recommend you learn to "ride the wave" and develop your problem-solving skills so you can build a healthy lifestyle (rather than trying to control your weight.)

Picture this: The lake of your life is fluid. The water swirls and has waves. Real things happen, things over which you have no control. However, you have your handy dandy surfboard (your problem-solving skills) and you learn to ride the waves of life. Sometimes you are up. Sometimes you are down. Usually you stay on the board and stay on top. Sometimes you get dumped into the water. Using your problem-solving skills that you have practiced a thousand times, you climb back onto your surfboard and get ready for the next wave.

Sometimes this is a difficult process. Often this is actually fun. **You put your energy into problem solving, NOT controlling.** This is an effective use of energy. It prepares you for the uncertainties of life. It leaves energy available to enjoy yourself. If you are tempted to seek control, remember the exhausting effort that goes into trying to keep the lake of life frozen. Don't try to freeze the water. Instead, polish your surfboard of problem-solving skills and "ride the wave"!

Guilt vs. Healthy Regret

I come from an Irish Catholic family. Debate or discussion was a primary recreation for us. When I was a teenager, I remember sitting by and listening to my brother and my father talk about guilt. "If people did not feel guilty about doing bad things, they would have no motivation to stop doing bad things." I knew most people would agree with their statement, yet I could FEEL something was wrong. As the years went by, I came to understand one of the problems with guilt.

Guilt makes people feel bad. Nobody wants to feel bad. In order to avoid feeling bad, people often numb themselves or tune out. For example, if you felt guilty about eating cookies, but part of you really wanted to eat the cookies, you might just eat the cookies and tune out while you are eating. Did you ever find yourself eating the last cookie and wonder where the rest of the package had gone?

Guilt makes people feel bad. Feeling bad about yourself reduces the motivation to do anything. Guilt about unhealthy eating or missing a workout may actually CAUSE you to stop trying to take care of yourself. Feeling bad can make you feel hopeless. "Oh, well, I already blew it. I am such a screw up. What's the use?"

If guilt doesn't help, what are we supposed to do when we mess up? I would like to introduce a concept that I call "healthy regret". When you do something that you wish you had not done, instead of beating yourself up with guilt, you could look at the situation differently. You could cultivate a healthy regret for your actions: " I wish I had not done that." Implicit in healthy regret is a wish for and the beginning of change. There is no self-deprecation, no internal name-calling. There is simply an awareness of a wish that things were different, a wish that things were better. THAT sounds like the beginning of a motivation for change. This awareness is necessary in order to make a plan to do things differently next time. When next you do (or don't do) something you regret, you can put your energy into doing (or not doing) better the next time. You can think of ways to succeed in the future, instead of beating yourself up with guilt for the past.

Prepare Tonight for Tomorrow

Getting started is tough. It is tough to start exercising. It is tough to start a different way of eating. It is tough to start any new habit. Heck, sometimes it is tough to start to get out of bed! Why is getting started so difficult? There are probably lots of reasons. One of the major reasons is inertia. *A body at rest tends to stay at rest.* Sitting on the couch tends to encourage sitting on the couch. One sedentary day tends to lead to the next. Ordering pizza tends to encourage ordering pizza. You get the idea. If getting started is so difficult, what can be done to make it easier?

Yes, a body at rest tends to stay at rest. However, the opposite is also true:

A body in motion tends to stay in motion.

We can use that fact to increase the chance that we will succeed in our self-care plans. You might try this: tonight, take a bit of time to prepare to take better care of yourself tomorrow. If you plan to go for a morning walk tomorrow, tonight you could set out your walking clothes and shoes. If you want to eat a healthier lunch tomorrow, tonight you could gather the ingredients for lunch in one spot or pack your lunch. If you plan to call a friend you haven't talked to for a while, you may put the phone number and a favorite mug by the phone to remind you to sit down and have a cup of coffee or tea with your friend.

Before you can be successful with this evening preparation for your next day, you have to tune into your own biorhythms. You cannot force yourself to prepare for tomorrow at a time in the evening when you are exhausted. Think about your evening energy. When, in your evening, do you have the best energy for this kind of planning and preparation? For some people it will be right when they get home from work, like a ritual to end one workday and aim for the next. Some people would hate that timing. Perhaps your biorhythms indicate that you should use your preparation for tomorrow as part of your bedtime routine. This may help you relax before bedtime. Or this might make you start thinking about tomorrow and get stressed. You need to tune in to yourself and figure out what works best for you. We are all so different. You need to really notice how you feel. Experiment and assess the results of your experiments until you find the best time in your evening to get ready for tomorrow. Choose a time to implement your evening preparation when it will be a helpful, not a hurtful, part of your evening. When you find the right time, you will be more likely to prepare tonight for tomorrow's activities.

Once you have set out your shoes, or packed your lunch, or found your friend's phone number, or whatever … what does that give you? Now you are in the **middle** of accomplishing your task or goal for tomorrow. **You have already started!** Now you are a body in motion, and you will tend to stay in motion. All you need to do is continue with what you have already begun and you will succeed at taking better care of yourself tomorrow.

Another Key to Success: Dynamic Flexibility

Let's say you have really decided to change your sedentary, unhealthy lifestyle. You have your plan. You are going to walk a mile every morning. Or you are going to eat five servings of fruits and vegetables every day. Yes, you have your plan. However, plans like the ones mentioned here don't leave much "wiggle room". One mistake, one off day, and you have failed.

**If your plan is static and rigid,
you are very likely to end up feeling like a failure.**

Life happens. Unforeseen circumstances pop up. When you make plans that have room for change, then you have room to make choices that work for you and your life. Your plans for improving your healthy lifestyle (or any other plans) must be able to fit into your life. Plans must be able to change. I call this dynamic flexibility (meaning to change and to bend.)

**Plans with dynamic flexibility are
the most likely to lead you to success.**

Let's look at the first example mentioned above and see how we might construct a goal with dynamic flexibility. The original rigid goal was that you planed to walk a mile every morning. When you implemented this goal, it might have unfolded like this: You got up and walked briskly for the entire mile on the first morning. You got sore muscles and had a slight limp the next day. If you were to stick to your static and rigid goal, you would have to force yourself to walk the entire mile on day two. You may have "walked off" the soreness as your muscles warm and you may have been fine. OR, you may have been developing an overuse injury. That is the physical side of the situation. What about your feelings and your attitude? Pushing yourself regardless of how you feel may cause you to hate walking. Hating walking would be the surest way to stop walking. Pushing yourself toward a goal that does not work for your body or your life leads to trouble.

If you were to design your walking goal with dynamic flexibility, it might look like this:

- I plan to walk three to five days this week.
- Today I will look at my schedule and decide what time of day would be best to walk tomorrow, or if I need a day off.
- Each time I walk, I will tune in to how I feel and choose a speed that varies between comfortable and challenging.
- If I did not walk yesterday, I will walk today.

This plan has room for you to live your life **and** you still have structure. You maintain your commitment to your walking goals.

You are fitting the plan into your life,

not trying to force your life into a rigid plan.

This goal does have structure. It also changes and bends as needed. This is an example of a dynamically flexible goal.

Let's try another example. Committing to eat five fruits and vegetables every day is a solid goal. It may also be a rigid goal because it does not have much flexibility in it. In order to succeed at this goal you would have to put substantial time and focus on eating and planning. You may be able to focus on eating fruits and vegetables some days. But as soon as you had a day when you were too busy to cook, or didn't have food in the house, or just plain did not like to eat fruits and vegetables, you would have failed at your goal. Often, feeling like a failure causes people to give up on a particular goal.

How would your healthy eating goal look if you were to change it to a goal with dynamic flexibility?

- I will buy more fruits and vegetables when shopping.
- I will order more salads, vegetables as side dishes, and fruit for desert, when I am eating out.
- I will try new ways to enjoy fruits and vegetables when possible.
- Each week I will select a meal and experiment with ways to enjoy more fruits or vegetables at that meal.

When you work toward these goals, you **will** be eating more fruits and vegetables. You will succeed at your healthy eating goal. Depending on your present lifestyle, you will probably work your way up to five a day within a few weeks or months. So what if the change is gradual! Gradual changes are so comfortable that you will be more likely to sustain the new behaviors. During all this time, you **ARE** succeeding at working toward your goals. You simply adjust your goals and continue to work on them. You continue to succeed.

**When your life gets hectic,
you do not have to abandon these goals that
change and bend with your needs.
Choosing goals with dynamic flexibility
sets you up for success.**

Procrastination

As I was writing this book, I kept putting off writing this section. I am not kidding. I am not making this up. I would scroll down the manuscript, see this section in red (which meant it was not finished yet), and then I would scroll right past. I did this at least fifty times! Then I said to myself, "this must be an opportunity for me to further explore the nature of, and possible solutions for, procrastination!" (Did you notice how I did not beat myself up, how I saw this as an opportunity to learn? I really do practice the skills I teach.)

Procrastination is a complicated topic. There are entire books dedicated to this one subject. I include this topic because procrastination is often one of the problems that gets in the way of healthy living and self-care. I want to give you three ideas to help reduce procrastination.

1.) "Just Start"

Tell yourself to "Just Start". This concept is quite different than the usual message we have been taught to give ourselves. You know the phrase: "Just Do It™". That sneaker slogan is very familiar. Many people use this concept to force themselves to accomplish goals and tasks in their lives. If you use this concept, you will have a tendency to think of the *entire* task:

- For exercising: You tend to think of doing your entire workout.

- For walking: You tend to think of the entire mile or two.
- For cleaning: You tend to think of cleaning all the drawers, the entire room, or the entire house.

There is a real problem with "Just Do It™".
This type of thinking can CAUSE procrastination.

It is intimidating. Where will you ever find the time when you will be able to do the entire task? Even if you find the time, where will you get the energy for it all? I have a better phrase for you to tell yourself:

"Just Start!"

There is a big difference between getting yourself to DO a task and getting yourself to START a task. It only takes a moment to start. You only need a little energy to start. It is not intimidating to "**Just Start**". It is just a little thing.

- "Just Start" your workout. Dress, pop your video in the player, and warm-up. That's all. Just start. Commit to starting, and you will probably enjoy doing the rest of your workout after you have started.
- "Just Start" your walk. Get dressed and do the warm-up for your walk. The momentum will probably carry you through the rest of your walk.
- "Just Start" your cleaning. Pull out one drawer, or one closet, or one corner. Just clean that. You may choose to clean something else after that.

There is one important condition when you commit to "Just Start":

After you "Just Start",
you MUST give yourself
permission to keep going
OR to stop.

I know. This sounds backward. However, if you always force yourself to keep going, then starting is the same as doing the entire task. You will find that you end up with the same resistance you had to forcing yourself to do the entire task. And that would be reasonable. If you always finish the task once you start, then "Just Start" would have turned into "Just Do It™". It seems odd to say giving yourself permission to *stop* doing the task will help end procrastination. But it is true. Take the pressure off. Once in a while let yourself stop after the warm-up, sometimes go home after only a few blocks, or only clean one small area and be done.

When you can choose to do the entire task
OR just do part of it, then you are free to "Just Start".
When you "Just Start", you just ended procrastination.

2.) Dangle a carrot or fill your gas tank, whichever works for you.

There are an infinite number of tasks to be accomplished in one's life. Luckily, if you are creative, there are also an infinite number of enjoyable or rejuvenating activities too. It seems that a key to reducing stress is to balance these two types of activities. It is best if there are some tasks and some enjoyable activities in each and every day.

OK, that seems simple enough. But once again, it is not as simple as it may seem at first glance. I challenge you to build a quality list of enjoyable and rejuvenating activities. All too often, we end up using "tune-out" activities, like watching TV and eating, when we need a break from the tasks of life. Instead of really enjoying ourselves or really rejuvenating, often we just tune out and procrastinate on the tasks of life.

A common reaction to this procrastination is to PUSH yourself to stop procrastinating. I never find pushing to be as effective as pulling. I encourage you to PULL yourself to do the tasks in your life by having more quality in your enjoyable and rejuvenating activities. Here is how it works.

Find activities to do that you really enjoy, activities that really make you feel better and refreshed. Then, you have two ways you can use these activities. You will find that sometimes it is better to use one way, other times you will be more effective using the other.

- **Dangle a carrot.** Tell yourself that you will do the task FIRST, and then you will really be able to enjoy your next activity. After your task has been completed, you will really appreciate the rejuvenating/refreshing activity. Use the fun or relaxing stuff (that you will do after your work) as a carrot to dangle in front of yourself as motivation to accomplish the task. Pull yourself to get the task done because you look forward to the enjoyable or rejuvenating activity you will do afterward.
- **Fill your gas tank.** Choose to do the rejuvenating activity first, before your task. Sometimes that is exactly what you need. Instead of constantly pushing and resisting the pushing, you can change your approach to tasks. Include some activity that will help you to feel better as a prelude to doing the task. In effect, you have put "feeling better" on your list of tasks. Then the second item on that list is the job or task (that you would have delayed starting for much longer.) This is like filling your tank before you get going. It can be very effective at reducing procrastination. The act of filling your tank is actually part of the trip. In a way, you have already started. You are not procrastinating.

I find a key to reducing procrastination is to gearshift between these two tools. There will be times when it is simply more effective to do the task first and enjoy or relax afterward. This is especially true if the task hanging over your head gives you stress. In that case, you need to do the task first to feel your best. If however, you are truly out of gas, then filling your tank may be the best choice. Only you can tell. You are the only real expert on yourself. You have the right to experiment freely with both of these tools. Try dangling the carrot. Notice how you feel. Try filling your gas tank. Notice how you feel. You will gradually gain skill at deciding which tool is the right one to use at any given moment. Give yourself permission to solve the problem of procrastination in the way that works for you. You don't have to push yourself with a feeling of "should" or "ought to". You are entitled to do what is best for you.

3.) Add one more client to the list of those who deserve your attention.

Doing things for your family, for your job, for your community, for your friends, for your church, etc. is commendable. It is good to do these things. When you think of it, each of us is like the executive who manages the departments of our lives and who has many clients. I have a proposal for you. In order to reduce procrastination, add one more client to your list. Yes, that is what I said. I want you to ADD another client to your already overloaded client list. As a matter of fact, I encourage you to add this client and put this client right at the top of the list because this is your most important client. Without the good health and well being of this client, everybody else on your list will not get the proper attention either. Have you guessed yet? Do you know who this new client is? Yes, I want you to add <u>yourself</u> to your list of clients.

I am not encouraging selfishness. I do not want you to ignore your other clients. I simply want you to add a client. If a family member, or co-worker, or neighbor, or friend, or church member, or someone else needed to be added to your list, you would do it. Well, I am telling you that there is someone who *desperately* needs your attention. It is your new client, your most important client. It is you.

Oftentimes it is not truly procrastination that stops us from doing the tasks in our lives. Sometimes it is that our priorities keep us running in so many directions that we could never accomplish all that we expect of ourselves. Sometimes we are drained dry from all the demands of tending others. I propose that you reduce procrastination by putting yourself at the top of the list of people who deserve your attention. Do the things that YOU need to get done. Feel your own accomplishments. Schedule in your own enjoyment and rejuvenation activities so that you will keep your gas tank full. (Interestingly, this will help rejuvenate you and end up allowing you to have more energy and attention to give to others in the long run.)

These may be some unusual ideas for reducing procrastination. Good. New ideas have a good chance of making a difference. In summary, to reduce procrastination, try these:

1.) Just start!
2.) Dangle a carrot or fill your gas tank, whichever you need.
3.) Add one more client to your list: that client is YOU.

Remember, you choose. You experiment. You assess the effectiveness of your choice. If it worked, enjoy. If your choice did not work, just try again with another choice!

The Compliment That Hurts

My mother wore the same suit to every one of her class reunions. I don't mean the same style suit. I mean the *same* suit. I remember that she always looked so pretty when she got dressed and went to the party. She was very proud to fit into the same suit every five years for each reunion. She did not stay the same size between reunions though. In real life, she fluctuated between a size twelve and a size twenty. Months before each reunion she would "buckle down", lose "the weight" until she "looked good", and fit into her black suit again. She was proud of her accomplishment. After all, so many of the "girls" really "let themselves go" over the years.

My mother had four daughters. We heard her friend's reactions to her many weight loss "successes". "Oh, Jeannie, you look wonderful!" "You look much better now." "You were really starting to look awful there for a while." As young girls listening to these conversations of the women around us, we learned these hurtful lessons that caused problems for all of us later in life: When someone loses weight, that is always a good thing. Thinner people look better. Anyone can, with enough willpower, lose weight anytime they want to. These were hurtful lessons. And these lessons were untrue.

Two of Jeannie's daughters were short and chubby. We learned that our bodies were unacceptable when we heard the grown-ups talk. Two other daughters were tall and lean. They also learned to criticize and measure their bodies. We were all in training for a lifetime of body loathing. Our teachers were the adult women in our lives. They did not mean to hurt us. These women were just doing what they were taught. Still, listening to these hurtful compliments wounded each of Jeannie's daughters.

Mom was wounded too. Every compliment about her brief thinness was also a criticism of her usual plumpness. Every compliment would come back to haunt her when her weight returned, as it always did.

No, I am wrong. Eventually, my mother did lose weight and keep it off. She did finally get off the diet and weight gain merry-go-round. When she was fifty-two years old, she was diagnosed with lung cancer. As the cancer ravaged her body she got thinner and thinner. One day, when I was visiting during her illness, we went to the corner shopping center. We ran into one of mom's old friends. I remember her friend saying, "Jeannie, you look great. You are so nice and thin!" A few weeks later, we all went to my sister's opera performance. Mom wore a beautiful gray slinky dress. I remember her saying, "One nice thing about having cancer is that I don't have to worry about my weight. I finally look good in these fitted clothes." A few months later she looked good in her casket too. All her friends said so.

The Little One Inside

For many people, it is easier to take care of others than it is to take care of themselves. If this is true for you, you may find this next concept helpful to you: ADD yourself to the list of people who deserve your care and tending. I am not saying that you should care less about other people. I am saying that you should **also** care about yourself.

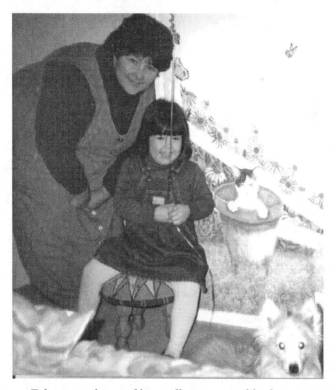

Take care of yourself as well as you would take care of a little one in your care.

I would like you to imagine some time in your life when you were in charge of taking care of a child. You may have had full-time responsibility, or you may have been tending this little one for the day. Would you let the little one who was in your care ...

- You would <u>not</u> let the little one stay up late at night even when you know exhaustion will follow tomorrow?
- You would <u>not</u> let the little one sit on the couch all day staring at the TV or the computer without moving for hours at a time?
- You would <u>not</u> let the little one remain isolated without playing with friends for long periods of time?
- You would <u>not</u> let the little one eat "entertainment foods" all day without enough food for fuel and nutrition?
- You would <u>not</u> let the little one avoid drinking water, in order to avoid trips to the bathroom?

Of course you would not let a little one in your care do all these harmful things.

You would make sure that the little one you were watching ate well and drank enough water, got enough rest, ran around and played enough so they wouldn't be fidgety, and enjoyed a stimulating environment (including play time with friends.)

What if you were just in charge of watching a little dog for the week? Yes, even the dog would get the food he needed, plenty of water and regular exercise in the yard or on a walk. The dog would be given things to play with so he wouldn't get bored and get into trouble. You would give the dog attention and affection.

These are basic needs of all creatures, big and small. Yet, very often, we do not even meet our own very basic needs. There are very good reasons why this happens. The reasons are different for everybody. I encourage you to explore within yourself the reasons that you sometimes don't take care of yourself. This can be a long process. Some people use therapy sessions, self-help books, and conversations with friends, etc. It can be hard work to understand yourself. It is worth the work. However, there is a way to encourage self-care, even before you have unraveled the deep psychological reasons it can be difficult. When I thought about the way people take care of little children and pets, I got an idea.

You may find it valuable to picture a little one *inside* of you. This little one has the same color hair as you have. His/her little face has big round eyes the same color as yours. This little one is probably even cute and chubby like a cherub (You know the kind. You just feel like hugging them and squeezing their fat little thighs. I digress. I like cherubs.) Well, now that you have pictured this little one inside of you, when you make choices on how to take care of yourself, how to talk to yourself, and what to think about yourself, consider the little one inside.

Take care of the little one inside of you.
Give him/her all the things necessary
to thrive and feel well:

- Eat healthy foods because they make you feel better.
- Enjoy entertainment foods occasionally, but primarily rely on your life to really meet your needs.
- Give yourself the water your body needs, even if this adds extra trips to the bathroom (that is just another opportunity to get moving!)
- Sleep as much as you need so you feel rested
- Enjoy your friends. Whether you engage people face to face, on the phone, or in a chat room, find people with whom you feel accepted and connected.
- And finally, get out and play! Move your body in some way that you enjoy. Feel your body's strength and flexibility. If you don't know any type of movement that is fun for you, take action to discover what activity you can enjoy.

Yes, these are the basic needs of all creatures great and small. These are YOUR basic needs. Sometimes life has taught us to ignore our own needs. It may be helpful to remember the little one inside of you. The little one (who you used to be) is still part of the grown up you. The little one inside of you deserves to have his/her basic needs met. The little one inside of you deserves good nutrition, fun activities, and to be appreciated body and soul (especially by you).

Kids Hear What You Say, and They Believe It!

I write this section for talk show hosts, newscasters, parents, teachers, coaches, doctors, and anyone who speaks where children can hear you. If you are a public figure or a role model for kids, it is especially important for you to be aware of this concept:

**Kids hear what you say about yourself,
and they learn to say the
same kinds of things to themselves.**

Watch the news. Most of the time when a reporter does a story about body size, weight, plastic surgery, or looks in general, the reporter adds a disparaging comment about their own body. A tiny female reporter on the morning news talks about her fat thighs. A prominent reporter who is thin comments "I'm not as thin as I should be." Reports on liposuction, stomach stapling, and tummy tucks, sound more like infomercials than news stories.

The media is supposed to present the facts about the news of the day. Instead, our kids are bombarded with body loathing comments and emotions. This damages all of us. But it especially damages children and teens.

**When you make body loathing
comments about your body,**

**you are teaching young people
to hate their bodies too.**

Every time you say that your butt is too big or your arms are too flabby, you are planting the seeds of body loathing in everyone who heard, especially the kids. Listen to what you say. Kids hear what you say about yourself and they believe it. Notice how often you make negative comments about your looks, or size, or hair, or whatever. If you continued to do this, YOU would be teaching the children who hear you to do the same.

**Make a promise to yourself NOW.
Make a promise to the children who hear you.**

**Stop saying negative things about your body.
Kids will follow your lead.
You can lead them well.**

Do It for the Children

If sometimes you feel bad about your body and you make negative comments about your body in public then you are having an effect on the people around you … some of those people are children. If self-acceptance and healthy living are very difficult problems for you, you may find motivation from this awareness. Think about the children in your life.

Are you a mom, dad, aunt, uncle, teacher, coach, nurse, doctor, or friend to a child? Are you a public figure who children can see or hear in the media? Then the way you think, what you say, how you live, affects the children in your life too. Perhaps you can find some motivation to take better care of yourself because it will help them.

As stated in the New England Journal of Medicine, in the January 1998 issue, "anorexia and bulimia are epidemic in this population -- and dangerous, with a mortality rate as high as twenty percent. Although many girls caught up in these practices are well aware of the hazards they would rather risk death than fall short in their attempts to attain the contemporary esthetic "ideal" of extreme thinness".

Anorexia is the most fatal of all the mental illnesses. Yes, more people die from anorexia than from any other mental illness. Bulimia destroys the digestive tract, the teeth, and can cause fatal heart arrhythmia. Compulsive overeating is often the result of restrained eating involved in dieting behaviors. With an awareness of the pain and suffering that can be triggered by dieting, you probably wish that future generations could be spared the pain of body loathing and eating disorders.

For many people who have battled their weight all their lives, the fear that a child who they care about may suffer from an eating disorder is very real. When a child gets an eating disorder, it is not the "fault" of the adults in his/her life. Eating disorders are complex, and your role as an adult who affects the child is just one of many factors. Yet the question remains: "What can I do, as a parent, an aunt, a teacher, a coach, a nurse or doctor, to decrease the likelihood that the child I care about will suffer body loathing and eating disorders?"

You can do plenty. You can either contribute to the problem or the solution. The choice is yours. I will mention some common sense steps you can take. These steps are not simple to implement, but your efforts will be worth it for you and the children you affect. There are volumes written on the subject of eating disorders and body dissatisfaction. Here are some thoughts and suggestions I can offer:

1.) Pay attention to your own behaviors, attitudes, and feelings about food and body image.

Clean up your own act. Kids learn from what you DO more than what you say. Begin eating for health, NOT to change your body size. Enjoy regular exercise because it is fun and feels good, NOT to shape your body.

2.) STOP making negative comments about your own body or other people's bodies.

Learn self-acceptance and body size-acceptance. This is a difficult process, but it is worth your effort for yourself and your children. As you go through the process of healthy living at your size, the children in your life will learn that process from you!

3.) Don't let fat jokes go unchallenged (you would not let racial or religious slurs go unchallenged.)

Speak up to the kids in your life. Speak up in front of the kids in your life. Write letters together to TV shows and advertisers who make fun of fat people. The media exalts thinness and portrays fatness as horrible, funny, and disgusting. Children who succumb to eating disorders and body loathing have come to believe these narrow stereotypical portrayals and will do harm to themselves in order to attain the "ideal" body size and avoid fatness. Teach the kids in your life that people of all sizes deserve respect. You will be teaching them to love and respect themselves, whatever body size is natural for them.

4.) Teach children to appreciate the beauty in diversity.

We can be part of redefining beauty for children, appreciating all sizes, all ages, and all ethnicities. This leaves room for children to appreciate themselves, whatever size, age, or ethnicity they are.

5.) Take a look at your own heritage. Preserve the healthy eating and self-acceptance that has been passed down to you. Let go of the negative attitudes about body size.

Children of different ethnic backgrounds have different views toward food, eating, and body image. Be active in promoting the positive attitudes toward people of all sizes that are present in your ethnic group. Notice the hurtful behaviors and fat-phobic attitudes that you have inherited also. Be active in letting go of these negative attitudes about fatness.

6.) Now, take a look at other ethnicities.

In some ethnic cultures, there are attitudes and norms that promote self-acceptance and self-esteem. When both large and small body size are accepted within an ethnic group, then people of all sizes can feel accepted. This is very helpful in the development of self-esteem.

Work toward adopting these helpful attitudes and norms. When you and the children in your life embrace the diversity of other people and customs in the world, you teach children an expanded worldview. They will learn to appreciate the differences in people and the value of uniqueness. They will be less likely to fall victim to the tyranny of thinness or any one "ideal" of beauty.

Just as there are different attitudes toward body size, there are different foods and attitudes toward eating in different ethnic groups. Which foods are more nutritious? Which attitudes are more self-accepting? Explore and enjoy the helpful attitudes and foods with the children in your life. Talking is good. Learning is better. Go to the library and attend fun cultural events. Doing is even better. You and the children in your life can plan and cook foods that other people enjoy. Experiencing diversity teaches acceptance of the uniqueness in other people.

**When uniqueness is valued,
children have more room
to value what is special and unique
about themselves,
including their body size.**

**This boils down to a few basic actions to help kids feel
better about themselves:**

- **Clean up your own act. Change your mind about
  body size and beauty. Kids can tell what you really
  think.**
- **Live a healthy lifestyle and take actions to end body
  loathing in your life and in the world. Kids learn
  from what you do more than from what you say.**
- **Expand your view of beauty to include all sizes, ages,
  and ethnicities. Kids learn their aesthetics from their
  environment.**

Appreciating diversity lets children have room to
appreciate themselves as unique individuals. Help children
experience eating and attitudes outside of your usual patterns.
Expand children's choices for healthy foods and new
attitudes about body image.

These are just some ideas for the prevention of eating
disorders. There are many ways to approach this important
topic. None of this is simple. Some of it is fun. All of these
processes are worth your time and effort. The payoff is not
only a healthier you, but children who are less likely to
develop eating disorders and more likely to feel good about
themselves.

Self-Care Heals Past Wounds

An important psychological effect of your self-care is that
you can FEEL that you have put yourself at the top of the list
of those who receive your care and tending. When you tend
yourself in your present day life, you help to heal yourself
from past emotional wounds. Everyone, no matter what kind
of childhood they lived through (even an "ideal" childhood

like those in storybooks), has had times when they were hurt because they experienced unmet needs. Some were lost in a crowd of a large family, some had parents who worked all the time, some just needed more attention, and some suffered abuse. These experiences result in emotional wounds. In your past, the person who was responsible to take care of you sometimes neglected or hurt you.

**In the present YOU are responsible
to take care of you.**

**How you treat yourself NOW
will either continue the cycle of hurt,
or will promote the cycle of healing.**

You have the choice to continue life with unmet needs and continue to hurt yourself, OR you can choose to tend and care for yourself and heal. You can heal past wounds by giving yourself what you need, by taking care of yourself.

**Every time you nurture yourself
by meeting your basic needs,
you heal yourself a little bit from past neglects.**

As you go through this process of building a healthy life for yourself, you are doing much more than improving your health. You are putting yourself at the top of the list of those who deserve your care. You are experiencing that *you* deserve your care. Good for you!

Chapter Two

Making Peace With Food

A Journey

The town of Lenni, PA was so small there was really no main street. There was just Lenni Road. It was more of a roller coaster than a road. It twisted and turned. It had a steep hill, and then a drop so steep that you actually rose up out of your seat briefly as the car descended. And then, there were the railroad tracks. When you went over the tracks the car and the passengers were shaken and bounced.

We drove up and down Lenni Road every day for almost two decades. The kids and I were on our own. When I was married, my husband traveled a lot. When they were nursery school age, they would giggle as they jiggled over the railroad tracks. They would gasp as they crested the hill and plunged into the steep descent. We liked the roller coaster road. We laughed.

On this particular journey, back in the early 1980s, it was just my husband and I. As we rode down Lenni Road, I was enjoying the ride more than usual because I was the passenger instead of the driver. I giggled and held my jiggling belly and breasts as we went over the railroad tracks. I bounced as we went over the hill and down. I was having fun until I noticed my husband's face. "What's wrong?" I asked. His comments appalled me (Which was a good thing, if I had agreed with him my self-esteem would have been badly damaged.) He said: "That's disgusting. You are so fat that you are like a blob of Jell-O jiggling around in the seat next to me." I asked him why he would say something like that. He replied: "I have to tell you that you are fat. Otherwise, you might stay that way. How will you know that you have to change?" At the time I was a size 12. I rode silently for the rest of the journey. We were divorced a few years later.

That evening I wrote this poem when we came home from that critical car ride. I found it last year in an old journal. At first I thought the poem was about a young woman speaking to her critical husband. Then it hit me. This poem could also be MY BODY speaking to ME. Over the years I have journeyed through the experience and recovery from my eating disorders (bulimia, compulsive over-eating, and exercise bulimia.) It took me decades to learn what my body already knew. Yes, this poem *was* my body speaking to me. Would your body give the same message to you?

If your goal is to change me,
Then your efforts are bound for resistance.

But if your goal would be to love me …
Then I will enjoy your love and give you mine.

And from my love,
I will do what I can so that you might be more happy.

What makes this difficult is that
You must love me AS I AM.

For if you love me so that I will change,
Then your goal is to change me.

And your efforts are bound for resistance.
But if your goal would be to love me ...

Eating Too Little for Your Body's Needs

If you use *controlling* your intake of food as a way to meet your emotional needs, if you are or have been told you might be anorexic, I have a special caution for you. If you consistently eat so little food that you do not get adequate nutrition (no matter what your body size), please read the following cautions carefully ... and read them again often.

You REALLY need to pay attention to yourself. Listen to the expert on you. Listen to yourself. Notice what helps you to eat nutritiously and take better care of yourself. Notice what makes it more difficult to eat your nutritious foods. You will find some of the concepts and exercises in this chapter NOT useful to you. *If you are or might be anorexic, if you consistently avoid eating enough nutritious foods for your body's basic needs (no matter what your body size), do not use anything in this chapter that gets in the way of nutritious eating.* Use everything that helps you take care of yourself and fuel your body with food. You have the right and the responsibility to build a healthy lifestyle. You deserve it.

Eating Too Much
for Your Body's Needs

If you use eating food to meet your emotional needs and sometimes find yourself overeating until you are uncomfortable, you will find this section especially useful. You will find concepts and exercises that will help you take better care of yourself and eat in a healthier way. This is true regardless of your body size.

Listen to yourself. Notice what helps you to eat healthy foods and take better care of yourself. Notice what makes it more difficult to eat a comfortable amount of food. Use everything that helps you take care of yourself and fuel your body with food. You have the right and the responsibility to build a healthy lifestyle.

We have all learned to use eating to cope with emotions. From infancy when our crying is calmed with milk to adulthood as we watch TV commercials, we are taught that food will make us feel better. The truth is, sometimes it does, and sometimes it does not. In this book there are specific exercises (that are enjoyable) to help you understand if and how you use food to cope with your emotions. I do not suggest that you just stop using food by employing willpower to suppress this coping mechanism. That would leave you with an unmet emotional need. That would cause problems in some other way. Instead, I encourage you to develop other coping mechanisms so that you CAN meet your needs better, in ways that are more effective than food. Then you will not only have a better relationship with food, you will have a life that works better for you. You deserve it.

A Gateway to Eating Disorders

Why am I talking about eating disorders in the chapter on your relationship with food? Because "watching your weight" or dieting ARE gateway behaviors to eating disorders. Not everyone who diets gets an eating disorder. However,

ALMOST EVERYONE WHO HAS AN EATING DISORDER STARTED OUT BY DIETING!

If you have been on and off diets (any form of restricted eating) in your lifetime, that process has probably damaged you. You can improve your relationship with food.

**This chapter is about normalizing
your relationship with food,
NOT finding a better way to diet.**

In my local classes and on-line groups called Healthy Eating with Bliss ^{TM}, many people come to lose weight. Some of these individuals are anorexic or bulimic, some are compulsive overeaters, some just want to get off of the dieting and weight gain merry-go-round. We all work together. We work on feeling better about ourselves, taking care of our bodies and our emotions. My goal is to shift the focus away from weight and toward healthy living and self-care.

I encourage you to do everything reasonable to build a healthy lifestyle with a balance of good nutrition, emotional well being, and regular moderate exercise. I encourage you to work toward all these goals INDEPENDENT OF YOUR WEIGHT!

**When you have done everything
you can do that is reasonable, then
you have two choices:**

accept yourself and your body
OR
do something unreasonable.

If good nutrition and regular moderate exercise result in your body remaining heavier than your fantasy weight (or some weight on one of the many arbitrary charts), what else should you do? Should you exercise excessively? Should you eat less than a balanced healthy amount of food? NO!

Whether you are 98 lbs. or 398 lbs.,
you should NOT exercise excessively or
eat less than a balanced healthy diet.
That would be pathological.

Instead, you should live a healthy lifestyle,
let your body find its own natural size,
and appreciate yourself as you are.

Lessons from a
Bulimic and Compulsive Overeater

These are some of the things I learned as I recovered from my eating disorders.

- Whatever my body size and shape, I am entitled to take care of myself!
- My body deserves to be fed nutritious foods.
- My muscles and joints deserve the pleasure and benefits of regular movement.
- My basic human needs deserve to be met.

I made small doable changes in my life with a goal of taking care of myself. Those changes were more likely to be permanent than any grand sweeping changes ever could be.

Those small changes added up to a comfortable self-sustaining healthy lifestyle that met my physical and emotional needs.

When I made changes with a goal of weight loss, those changes were temporary. The very words, "on the program" and "off the program", implied that there was some "expert" telling me what to do or how to eat. There is nobody except me who can figure out what I should do and how I should eat in order to meet my unique set of needs. I need to TUNE IN so that I can learn from my experiences and make choices that meet my needs better.

The fact is that food *does* meet some of our physical and emotional needs. That is normal for all human beings. Food is supposed to be *one* way to meet our physical and emotional needs. There is a problem when we use food as the ***primary*** way to meet our needs.

> **The problem is not the food. The problem is that we spend too much time and energy eating (or not eating) instead of improving our lives. The problem is using food to tune out from how we feel and what we need.**

I kept asking myself two questions, "What do I need now?" and "What is the best way for me to meet that need?" I had to find out, through personal experimentation, what was right *for me*. No book, no program, no "expert", could tell me. I had to listen to myself and learn what I needed.

I wanted to improve my relationship with food, not to lose weight, but because food was not meeting my needs. I used my relationship with food as a tool to learn more about myself.

In order to understand what needs I was trying to meet with food, I decided to keep track of how I was feeling. (I had to avoid any behaviors that were similar to dieting behaviors. I would *not* write down what I ate.) Instead, *I would write down what I needed when I ate.* I found it most helpful to think and write down the need before I choose to eat. (After I ate, I often could not remember how I felt or what I thought.) Here are some of the needs I discovered:

- Fuel: I often ate because I was hungry and my stomach was growling.
- Entertainment: Sometimes food just tasted good and I wanted the pleasure of eating.
- Accomplishment: I could not face any other task, so fixing a nice meal met my need to accomplish something.
- Comfort: From mother's milk to chocolate cake, food has been and should be one possible source of comfort. It is just not the *only* source!
- Distraction: When I had an unpleasant feeling or thought, eating sweets would numb me.

This was educational, but it was only part of my question. I wanted to know what my needs were, and *if* my needs were being met when I ate. So, I took the time *before* I ate to write down what I needed. I took the time *after* I ate to notice how I felt. *Did eating meet that particular need?* If it did, I circled the need to symbolize a satisfied need. If it did not, I put an "X" through the need to symbolize an unmet need. When I reviewed my last week's record, I saw more "X"s than circles. I discovered many unmet needs that were hidden within my relationship to food.

Once I was more aware of my unmet needs, I got creative and found better ways to satisfy my needs. I used problem-solving to build a LIFE that met my needs. I chose to improve my relationship with food because I knew I deserved more satisfaction in my life. It had nothing to do with my weight. My weight was and must remain irrelevant.

Watching my weight and dieting were gateway behaviors to compulsive overeating and compulsive under eating and compulsive over-exercising. To recover from my bulimia I had to take the focus off of my weight. I recommend the same for you.

Don't do anything to lose weight.
Do everything to take care of yourself.
Don't watch what you eat.
Watch what you need.
Then, do everything you can to
meet your needs more effectively!

The Pink Elephant

I want you NOT to think about a pink ceramic elephant. Do NOT picture this twelve-inch tall elephant sitting on the table in front of you. Do NOT think of the lime green inside the ears or the cute little purple toenails. How are you doing? Are you NOT thinking about it? Of course you *are* thinking about it! That is all you can think about when I am commenting on it at length. It is impossible to NOT think about something. It is virtually impossible to NOT do something. Remember these characteristics of human thinking and behavior when you set your goals.

How many times have you tried not to eat this or that food? Instantly, all you can think of is the forbidden food. You experience powerful cravings. Trying not to eat makes you think about eating. I will never recommend that you NOT eat particular foods. You do not need the cravings. I will encourage you to eat more nutritious foods that you enjoy. That is something you can DO.

Have you ever tried to STOP being sedentary? Every time you notice yourself, you are sitting. It feels like you are doing the exact behavior that you wanted to stop. The truth is, you cannot stop sitting around. You can START moving a little at a time. You CAN take action. That is where you have power, in your actions. There is only frustration in trying to NOT do something.

Have you ever tried NOT to think critical thoughts? "I will stop criticizing my body." or "I will stop thinking I'm lazy." As you think of what kind of thoughts to avoid, *you are in the middle of thinking critical thoughts.* It is impossible to DO a negative! Instead, I will encourage you to consciously choose a more positive way of phrasing things in your own head and out of your own mouth. "I will appreciate my body." or "I will acknowledge the obstacles to accomplishing my goals." Practice choosing action (what you WILL do), instead of trying NOT to do something.

It takes every second of every minute of every hour of every day to NOT eat, or NOT criticize, or NOT anything. It only takes a moment to eat some healthy food, to appreciate yourself in some way, to get up and feel your body move. It only takes a moment to take an action or think a thought. This is your life. Instead of focusing on what you want to avoid, pay attention to what you want to add to your life. DO something. (By the way, I love pink elephants. I think about them all the time.)

Now and Later

When I stand up in front of a class full of lifelong dieters and tell them they will be working toward the goal of eating whatever they want, they look at me incredulously. Dieting, by its nature, means controlled eating and deprivation. Healthy Eating with Bliss™, by its nature means UNRESTRICTED eating where your *choices are made based on what you want.* Your new skills will be to experience what you eat more fully and to expand your awareness of what you want to include the present moment and the future. With this expanded awareness, *you tend to want healthier foods in more reasonable amounts.*

I use the phrase "now and later" to refer to:

1.) experiencing your eating now

2.) being aware of your how you will feel later

For example, when you sit down to eat a meal, you enjoy the flavor, aroma, and feel of the food as you eat. (Good! That is "savoring your food". It will be a tool you use in your journey toward healthy eating!) Later, after you eat, you will also feel the effects of your meal. You may feel comfortably full, or feel uncomfortably overstuffed. The choice is up to you. Do you want to enjoy your meal BOTH as you eat it AND afterward?

Learn about your body and your reactions to food. This is not easy. Life is so busy and complicated it is difficult to notice the connection between what we do and how it makes us feel later. This is a connection worth making. You can use writing to help you make this connection. I know, you may cringe at the thought of writing down what you eat. I will **not** suggest that you engage in this particular diet ritual. Most of us have been burned in the past by diet experiences that required writing down every bite of food eaten. That is why I suggest we do *not* focus on writing what you ate. The food is not the issue right now. Connecting to how food makes you *feel* is the issue.

I suggest you write down how you FEEL after you eat. Notice what you experience right after you eat.

- **Do you feel comfortable, like saying "Ahhhh" with a sigh of delight?**
- **Do you feel uncomfortably full and like groaning?**

Yes, I am focusing on physical feelings for now. I do that in order to avoid the guilt and judgment that may be included in emotional reactions to eating. What about your experiences in the few hours after you eat?

- **After your breakfast, notice how you feel mid-morning.**
- **After your day of meals and snacks, how do you feel in the evening?**

Be aware of your energy levels, your moods, your cravings, and whatever else you can notice. Now that you are tuned in to the effects of your eating, you may be more open to look at the cause. When you are ravenous by mid-morning, ask yourself, "What did I have for breakfast?" Was there some protein and heart healthy fat included? These are the foods that are used more slowly by the body and satisfy longer. When you feel compelling cravings for cookies, donuts, and other foods high in fat and sugar, notice what you have eaten in the hours and days before. Eating foods high in fat causes the neurochemical called "galanin" to be released. Galanin causes you to crave more fats! Believe it or not, this is good news. *This means that you have the power to affect your cravings.* You do not have to just cope with cravings. You can reduce cravings for fats later in the day by choosing certain foods lower in fat earlier in the day. What a wonderful gift to give yourself, wrestling with fewer cravings!

> **This is a fundamental shift in motivation. I do not recommend you eat less fat because you "should" or because you "ought to". I do not recommend that you eat less fat in order to lose weight.**
>
> **I recommend you give yourself a more peaceful evening with fewer cravings. It just happens that one way to give yourself this gift is to eat lower fat foods with better nutrition earlier in the day.**
>
> **Now you have a non-restrictive motivation. You are just giving yourself a nicer evening.**

Knowing how you react to foods will give you the awareness you need to choose to eat foods in the amounts that you can best enjoy "now and later". Do some foods make you feel lethargic? Then, don't eat them before a high-powered business meeting. However, you may consciously choose to eat a lethargy-inducing food when you want to chill out and do nothing for a while. After you eat some foods, do you have to cope with lots of cravings and urges to eat more, even though you are not really hungry any longer? Would you like to avoid having to wrestle with those cravings and urges? Then choose to avoid those foods! You are NOT restricting any type of food. You are giving yourself the gift of not having to wrestle with cravings!

Some Common Myths

Myth: You have the power to change your body weight as much as you want to, if you only try hard enough.

Fact: Permanent weight loss or gain is not under your control. You can <u>affect</u> your weight, not control it. Changes in your weight are the result of a complex combination of variables: dieting history, genetics, age, metabolism, health, lifestyle, and many more.

> **You do not have control of the many variables**
> **that affect your body weight; therefore**
> **you do not have control over your weight.**

Focus on your lifestyle choices instead of your weight. When you build a healthy eating style and exercise regularly you will find yourself at your natural weight. If you want to weigh less than your natural weight, you would have to do something obsessive or compulsive to maintain that unnatural weight.

Tip: Work on accomplishing goals of healthy eating and regular fun exercise, rather than a specific weight loss goal.
- Eat nutritious foods when hungry
- Stop eating when satisfied
- Meet your emotional needs without always using food
- Enjoy regular reasonable exercise
- Be patient and accept your body's own natural weight

******

Myth: When on any reasonable weight reduction diet, you can expect to lose one to two pounds a week.

Fact: Body weight changes at different rates for different people. Some people have a VERY efficient set point mechanism. They remain at a stable weight even with healthy lifestyle changes. Some people may lose a very small amount, ¼ pound a week. If weight loss were the goal, this would feel like a failure because it would not show up on most scales. It would be difficult to keep working so hard if nothing showed up on the scale. However, this small barely noticeable weekly weight loss, would result in a 13-pound weight loss per year. If you have an expectation of one to two pounds per week, you will probably be disappointed and get discouraged. *Weighing yourself can sabotage your attempts at healthy eating and exercise.* Sometimes all it takes is one trip to the scale to feel defeated and result in a binge. If you do not lose weight fast enough you may give up and stop taking care of yourself. You may respond in the opposite way. When you hit a "plateau", you may become excessively restrictive in your eating and/or overly rigorous in your exercise. These can lead to pathological behaviors. *A focus on weight loss often causes frustration and hopelessness or obsessive behaviors that can be unhealthy.*

Tip: Stop weighing yourself. Remember you can measure your success and appreciate your progress in much more effective ways. See the beginning of chapter one "Redefine

Success", for new ways to measure success. Try writing your accomplishments down in order to help you focus on your successes.

******

Myth: People who want a healthy lifestyle should not eat deserts, donuts, candy, etc.

Fact: A healthy lifestyle includes normal eating. Normal eating means that *sometimes* you eat just because food tastes good or feels good. If you rigidly restrict your eating and plan never to eat certain foods, you may be setting yourself up for a binge. I call foods that have little nutritional value but taste good "entertainment foods". Even people with a healthy lifestyle eat entertainment foods sometimes. This only becomes a problem when you use food as a *primary* source of entertainment or to meet other emotional needs.

Tip: Get in touch with WHY you are eating. Most people eat for comfort, reward, distraction, anger, relaxation, etc. When you choose food as your primary way to meet these needs, you are not only eating unnecessary food; you are missing the opportunity to do something more effective to meet your needs. **Make your own list of other ways to meet your needs. Do it now.** This is just an example to get you thinking:

- To comfort yourself: take a warm bath, walk in the garden, give yourself a hand massage with lotion.
- To reward yourself: go see a movie, buy something you have wanted (and can afford), put on some music and dance!
- For relaxation: take a walk in the park, go to a museum, soak your feet.
- To cope with anger: call an understanding friend, write a letter expressing your anger (Don't send it until you have cooled down. Only send it after you have edited out the cuss words.)

You get the idea. But here is the key. **You have to make up these lists ahead of time.** In the moment when you feel like using food to meet an emotional need, you may not be able to think of anything else. If you have the list made up ahead of time, you can use it and choose a non-food coping mechanism. You will rely on food less and you may even improve some things in your life too.

******

Myth: You should always resist cravings and remain in control of your appetite.

Fact: There are many reasons we crave certain foods. For example, women often crave chocolate as a result of hormonal changes in the monthly cycle. During that cycle, women experience different caloric needs. Some women require an increase of as much as 200 to 700 calories of food energy per day on certain days of their monthly cycle. For both men and women, it is not all in your head. Sometimes it is in the chemicals in your body. The neurotransmitter galanin causes a craving for high fat foods. Neuropeptide-Y causes you to crave carbohydrates. Your appetite is not flat and unchanging like a frozen lake. Your appetite is like the waves on the ocean. You cannot control them, but you can learn to ride them. When you get some skill, your appetite can become an asset rather than a liability.

Increase your awareness of your appetite. Play with it. When you eat a high protein meal, how long are you satisfied? When you eat sugars and fats, do you crave more of the same? If you skip breakfast and have a small lunch, are you ready to eat the house later that night? What are your trigger foods that make you want to eat more and more? Learn what makes it difficult and what makes it easier for you to <u>want</u> to eat nutritious foods.

Tips:

- When you have a craving, eat something healthy first. Wait a bit. You may not even have the craving any more. What if you still have the craving? Satisfy it. You will be able to be satisfied with less entertainment food because you have already eaten your nutritious food.

- Satisfy cravings with less fat and sugar if possible. Choose chocolate hard candies instead of milk chocolate. Hard candy lasts longer and has less fat. Try chocolate graham crackers instead of cookies. If this does not feel right for you, then don't do it. Listen to the real expert. That's you. When you choose to satisfy a craving, really taste what you eat. Savor it. Don't just sneak the food past your awareness and your taste buds by eating fast and unconsciously.

- Eat breakfast, lunch, dinner, and healthy snacks every day. When you concentrate on eating all that healthy food, you will not have as much room in your mind or your stomach for entertainment foods.

- Choose low fat foods early in the day and your brain will release less of the neurotransmitter galanin. You will experience less craving for fat in the evening.

- Savor your food, especially if you are eating to satisfy a craving. If you slip the food past your awareness and past your taste buds, you will have to eat much more to be satisfied.

- When the next bite is not as delicious as the last bite, why eat it? Remember that hunger is the best seasoning. **Don't waste your appetite on foods that are not nutritious or delicious.**

Your Motivation Matters

When it comes to making changes in yourself or your life, the reason **why** you make changes will have more to do with your success than anything else will.

Your motivation is the single most important factor in achieving and maintaining a lifestyle change.

Think of January, when New Year's resolutions are in the air. Think of spring as the beach season approaches. These are times when people often start a diet. You already know the end of that story. You have probably lived through it, or known someone who has. Most of the time, dieters do lose weight, only to regain the weight plus a few extra pounds within two to five years. How can you avoid this physically and psychologically damaging cycle? My answer may shock you.

Everybody knows the buzzwords; "Diets don't work." So, I will not say, "don't diet to lose weight". I will say:

"Don't do anything to lose weight."

Oh, my gosh! Did I really say that out loud? Yes, I did. And I will say it again. Please do not do *anything* to lose weight! Why would I say such a thing? Because,

If weight loss is the reason why you eat healthy foods and exercise, you will probably not continue healthy living activities if your weight fluctuates or plateaus … and weight ALWAYS fluctuates or plateaus.

If weight loss is your motivation, you are practicing and encouraging self-criticism. After investing in this negative motivation, you will be less likely to accept yourself even if you do lose some weight. You may find that you will cultivate a loathing for your fuller body as you quest for a smaller one.

**If weight loss were your primary goal,
then every workout would become an act of self-criticism.
If weight loss were your primary goal,
then every food choice would be based
on rejecting your body.
Every action would reinforce the hurtful message
that your body is wrong and deserves criticism.**

If you change your lifestyle in order to attain a certain size or shape, what will you do if your body does not cooperate? Imagine you just spent a year working hard to get into a pair of jeans you used to be able to wear. Imagine you exercised every day and ate nutritious foods so you could fit into those jeans. At the end of the year, if they fit, you would be a success. But, what if they didn't fit? What if, after everything, you were still not the "right size"? You would have worked for a year and failed at losing enough weight. You would very likely give up on your healthy lifestyle, because it did not work.

How many people do you know who struggle forever with "those last five pounds"? Sometimes they give up and abandon all efforts to exercise or eat healthy. Sometimes they redouble their efforts and become over-exercisers or obsessive dieters. Should a person cultivate obsessive behaviors, exercise several times a day, or eat less food than is reasonable? If a healthy lifestyle results in a plus-size body, should a person feel compelled to develop an obsessively-controlled lifestyle to be the "right size"? Isn't that pathological behavior? Wouldn't it be better if people worked on living healthy lifestyle and appreciating whatever size and shape body nature has given them?

When I say: " Don't do anything to lose weight", that is only half of my message. The other half is very important:

"Do everything you can to build a healthy

comfortable lifestyle and take care of yourself!"

Notice the beginning of this statement. Do what you can and appreciate whatever you do. You cannot fail at this goal. Whatever you weigh, whatever your fitness level, however you eat, you can work at improving your lifestyle.

**When building a healthy lifestyle is your primary goal,
EVERY ACT BECOMES
AN ACT OF SELF-NURTURING!
With every appreciative workout and
every nutritious meal, you heal
from the body-loathing that you have been taught.**

Well, actually, instead of <u>working</u> at building your lifestyle, I encourage you to <u>play</u> at improving your lifestyle. Notice the phrasing as I talk about the areas you might play with. I never use self-critical motivation. Instead, I focus on the positive reasons for making changes.

- You might choose to exercise more because you want to enjoy more flexibility, increased strength, or more stamina.
- You might enjoy more fruits and vegetables because of all the nutrients, fiber, and phytochemicals that improve your health.
- You may reduce your intake of sweets because you have more energy when your blood sugar is more level.
- If you eat when you are hungry, food will taste better and you will feel less deprived.
- If you stop eating when you are satisfied, you will be able to enjoy that feeling of comfortable fullness (ah, I like that feeling), and avoid feeling uncomfortably over-stuffed.
- When you use other skills and activities to cope with stress, fatigue, or anxiety, you may find that those skills and activities are more effective at fixing your life than food was.

When you make these changes in your lifestyle, your body will change. How will it change? Will you lose weight? I don't know. Your body weight and shape are determined by a complicated set of variables. You do not have control of all of those variables. I cannot predict the results of your lifestyle changes on your complicated body. I can tell you what I have seen as my clients build healthier lifestyles. I see people who feel better about their bodies, think less about food and enjoy nutritious eating more. I see increased self-confidence. People become more able (physically, mentally, and emotionally.)

Pay attention to how you talk to yourself. Notice *why* you make the choices in your life. When making choices, find motivations that are encouraging and appreciative. Eat healthy foods and exercise because you deserve to feel good *(not to lose weight.)* You will be happier today and more successful tomorrow. You will be successful at taking care of yourself and building a healthy lifestyle!

Mic Jagger Saved My Butt

I remember looking into the mirror and wondering how I got two black eyes. I had not been in a fight. I had not bumped into anything that I could remember. What could it be? Oh well, never mind. I went about my normal day. I ate lunch. I ate cookies. I ate popcorn. I ate brownies. Then I felt sick. So, I threw up. As I was rinsing my face off (and planning what I could eat next) I looked in the mirror again. My eyes weren't really black, they were maroon colored all around. At the edges I could see tiny little maroon dots. Then I realized that all these hundreds of tiny dots were broken blood vessels. These broken blood vessels were from throwing up, often six times a day. That was when I realized I was bulimic. That was back in 1978.

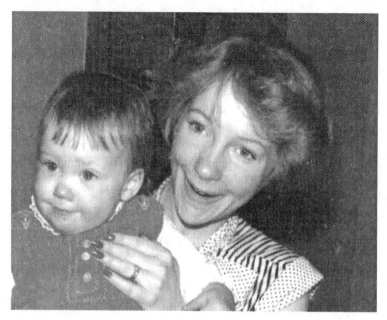

Me, my daughter, and my eating disorder

As I looked in the mirror, I asked myself, "Why did I do that? Why did I just throw up? Why did I *have* to throw up?" The answer was clear. After eating all that food, if I did not get rid of it, I would get fatter. At that time, I was terrified of gaining any weight. I believed that it was worth doing *anything* necessary to avoid gaining weight. I also knew that I could not stop myself from eating, despite all my willpower. Up until that moment, it seemed perfectly reasonable to "get rid" of the food I had eaten so I would not get fat. "Hmm ... something is *not* reasonable here." I have two black eyes and I'm throwing up all day. I know that bulimia can cause my heart to stop beating, blow out my esophagus, rot my teeth and leave me in dentures before age thirty. No, this is not reasonable, let me think about this.

I stood in my little yellow bathroom, wearing my red robe. I looked into the oval mirror for an answer. I knew there was a clue here, inside of me, if I could only listen well enough to my thoughts. I found two basic thoughts hanging in my mind: "I can NOT get fatter." "I am compelled to eat." At first it seemed there was no way to live with these two thoughts unless I did throw up. Then I decided to focus on one thing at a time. I started by focusing on my eating. I wanted to understand myself better. The answer must be INSIDE of me. A series of questions hit me: "What compels me to eat?" "What drives me?" "What am I looking for?" "What do I need when I eat?" "What do I want?" As I stood there I heard a voice in my head. The voice was deep and pulsing. I knew that voice. It was Mic Jagger who answered my questions. I am not kidding. In my head, I heard Mic Jagger singing: "Satisfaction ... satisfaction. I can't get no satisfaction."

I was looking for satisfaction. I was looking to eating to give me some kind of satisfaction. I tried something sweet. No, that was not it. I tried something salty. That did not satisfy me either. I tried crispy, smooth, and chunky foods. It felt like there was something here in this pantry that would do the trick. I just had not found it yet.

It never occurred to me that I should look into my LIFE instead of my pantry for satisfaction. At that time I was twenty-five. I had two children, ages one and three. I lived alone in a huge house with a huge yard in the middle of the woods, while my much older husband traveled on business six days a week. I thought I was a complete failure. I was fat. My husband constantly watched his weight and made sure that I knew I should too. He told me; "If I don't keep criticizing your fat ugly bulges, you might give up and stay this way." At the time I wore a size 14. I also thought I was lazy. Every other woman in the world could keep a clean house and mine was a constant mess. I only had two kids. My mom had seven kids and she kept the house clean. What the hell was wrong with me? My husband told me I reminded him of a sloth (that is an animal who hangs around doing nothing for so long that moss grows on him.) I could never finish the tasks on my list. I never stuck to an exercise program. I could not stop eating. Of course, at that time, I did not see any other problems except my food problem. If I only got this food thing under control, then everything in my life would be better. I continued my pathological focus on eating, food, and body loathing.

I kept eating one thing and then another, looking for satisfaction. When I wasn't satisfied, I had to "get rid" of the food. I had to "empty out". Isn't it interesting that I had all these euphemisms for throwing up? Before the morning when I noticed my black eyes, I had never even used the words "throwing up" in my mind. "Throwing up" was just too gross. Suddenly, on that morning, I realized that using these euphemisms was one way I was avoiding facing what I was doing to myself. I decided from now on to call a spade a spade. I was throwing up all the time. I wanted to stop.

**Since I was accustomed to focusing on my eating,
I used awareness of my eating
to help me stop overeating and throwing up.**

If I was looking for satisfaction when I ate, then by God, I would get satisfaction! I made a promise (actually it was a vow, I was raised Catholic after all) to myself that I would only eat something if it was absolutely delicious. If it was not absolutely delicious then I would not eat it. I was not going to spend any of the precious room I had in my belly on any food that was less than scrumptious.

I started really tasting my food. Yes indeed, I savored it. I noticed how the food looked. I set out nice place settings for myself when I ate. I took time to arrange the food on lovely plates. I looked at my food for a while before I ate it. (Note: If the food did not look delicious, I did not eat it. I was sticking to my vow!) Next, I appreciated the aroma of the food. Did this food smell delicious? If it did, I ate it. If it did not smell delicious, I did not eat it. How could something that does not smell delicious satisfy me? Once my food looked and smelled wonderful, I would take small bites so that the flavor would last longer. I savored each bite, giving it time to linger on all my taste buds. (Did you know that when you close your lips with food in your mouth and exhale you enhance the flavor of your food dramatically? Try it. It does!) I was very aware when I ate. When the next bite was not as delicious as the last, I did not eat any more. My only motivation was increased enjoyment of my food -- satisfaction. (I was NOT doing this to eat less or to lose weight. If those motivations crept in, I felt like throwing up again! I put great effort into focusing on the enjoyment of eating as my motivation.) I learned about a new pleasure as a result of this very conscious eating, the pleasure of finding that I was "perfectly full".

My eating habits changed dramatically. Not only did my cookies taste better, but I could only eat a few cookies before they lost their scrumptious flavor. I was not going to waste my appetite on any food that was less than delicious! I started eating more healthy foods too. This was amazing. There was no deprivation, no limitations. My only measuring stick was my own pleasure and enjoyment. I stopped eating a slice of pecan pie on the fourth bite … because it was not as delicious as the third bite! I was not going to waste my appetite on a bite that was not wonderful.

I vividly remember the first time I ate without wanting to throw up. It was two years after I had heard Mic Jagger's song in my head. This process was not quite as easy as it sounds. Of course I goofed up and ate more than I wanted at times. Sometimes, if I ate a bit more than was comfortable, I really wanted to throw up. I had to strongly remind myself that my body could handle what I had eaten. The world would not change because I was uncomfortably full.

I went from someone seeking satisfaction in eating to someone seeking satisfaction in "perfect fullness". What a change! Food became the tool I used to TUNE IN to how I was feeling. Food was not my anesthetic any more. I discovered a world of emotions and unmet needs. When the next bite was not as delicious as the last bite, I asked myself "Why eat it?" I got amazing answers. I wanted to eat food for comfort, distraction, reward, relaxation, adventure, rebellion, etc. As time went by, I realized eating more food would not really meet any of those needs, not in the long run. I decided to work toward finding more effective ways to meet my emotional needs. My focus changed. Eating, even when enjoyable, was not satisfying enough. I had to find satisfaction in my life. Now I had something to work on that would make a difference. I could work on what was really important. I could work on my LIFE, instead of my weight or my eating.

An Unusual Exercise

It is always so fun to watch the reactions of the people who have been dieting all their lives when I give this first "exercise" in my "Healthy Eating with Bliss^{TM}" classes and on-line groups. After years of thinking of food as "bad" and appetite as the enemy, this exercise is quite shocking. It is harder to do than you might think, but it is fun.

Savor

This is a tough exercise. At first it will seem simple. Usually it will be enjoyable. But it will still be tough. You will be surprised at your reaction when you try this. You may discover things about yourself and your feelings that you did not know. Your first eating exercise is:

**Whenever it
seems reasonable,**

SAVOR YOUR FOOD.

**Enjoy the aroma.
Appreciate how delicious it looks.
Really taste it.**

Swirl it around all your taste buds.

Experience it!

As you try this, you may find that you are more satisfied when you eat. You may be more satisfied with less food because you are really experiencing what you are eating. Most compulsive behaviors are about tuning something out. Often people eat to numb or distract themselves. This exercise is the opposite of compulsive eating. You are not tuning out. YOU ARE TUNING IN! This time, food is not an escape; it is a tool for self-discovery.

If it makes you more comfortable, you can also focus on noticing when the next bite of food does not taste as delicious as the last. At that point, when eating is not as enjoyable, you can ask yourself: **"Why eat any more?"** You may be surprised at your answer to this simple question. But, we will get back to that later.

Be patient, this is not easy. You will not savor your food all the time. Sometimes you will just scarf down a lunch because you are hungry and need to get back to work. That is fine. That is normal eating too.

M&Ms®

Lauren was not overweight (This is not her real name. I always change the names to preserve confidentiality.) She was an average-sized woman. We were working together in counseling to reduce her depression, increase her self-esteem, and improve her family relationships. She had trouble sleeping, felt lethargic (especially at home in the evenings), was quick to anger, and seemed to get sick all the time.

Of course we worked on many different aspects of her feelings, choices, reactions, motivations, etc. After a while, one issue surfaced that seemed as if it could have an effect on many of the other issues at hand. Resolving this one issue provided profound and immediate results. When we solved this one problem, Lauren slept better, had more energy in the evening, felt better about herself, and had more patience with her family in the evening. That is the story I want to tell you now. You may find it interesting. You may find yourself in the story. You may find new hope for coping with an old problem.

Lauren's days were very stressful. She was rushed in the morning. Getting herself and everyone else in the family out the door on time was a real challenge. There certainly was no time to sit down and have breakfast. Coffee to go, with cream and sugar, was all she needed to stave off hunger pangs. She drank lots of coffee all day long. At lunch, with everyone at work watching, she found it easy to eat a small reasonable lunch. She knew that no one approves of a glutton, so she ate a light lunch with all the other women at work. Then, she was back to coffee in the afternoon. She was busy from the moment her workday started until it ended and she was scheduled to head home and cook dinner for the family. By the time Lauren sat down in her car at 5:00 p.m. she was frazzled, starving, and exhausted.

She remembered ten years ago when it began. On the way home from work one day, she decided to stop at the convenience store to get a snack for the kids. She was REALLY hungry, but she was going home to eat right away. There was no need to buy real food now. The kids, however, would enjoy a snack with TV tonight. She went in and bought a family size bag of M&Ms … for the kids.

As she was driving home, she decided to have a few M&Ms. She set the bag in her lap, opened it, and popped a handful in her mouth. Her drive home was forty-five minutes long. As she pulled into her neighborhood, she was astonished to realize the family size bag of candy was empty. How did that happen? Oh, well, never mind. It will never happen again. But it did happen again. It happened every night for the last ten years. No matter how much willpower Lauren mustered, no matter how much she hated herself for it, she kept doing it. She kept buying and eating a family size bag of candy after work every day. After talking to many nutritionists, hypnotists, diet counselors, and such, she could not seem to stop eating M&Ms. All she wanted was to stop this behavior. She wanted me to help her stop eating M&Ms. My suggestion appalled her. However, after ten years of feeling like a failure, she was willing to try anything. What was my suggestion? What did I tell Lauren?

"Do not try to stop. If trying to stop eating has not worked for ten years, why should I recommend that you try the same ineffective solution again? This time, try something different to cope with your irresistible cravings for M&Ms. Taste them. Don't just shovel them into your mouth mindlessly because you don't want to notice what you are doing. Eat them one at a time, slowly. Let each one melt. Don't chew. When the candy is in your mouth, close your lips and exhale through your nose. (This drives the chocolate molecules to a sensory organ in the nose and increases sensation.) Notice how delicious the candy tastes. Now (this is the important part) when the next bite does not taste as delicious as the last bite, ask yourself a question: "Why eat it?"

You may find that you simply do not need to eat any more of that particular flavor or food because it is not as delicious anymore. Then you may be able to stop eating comfortably without a struggle. You might be satisfied.

You may also find an emotional answer to the question of "Why eat it?" If this happens, pay attention to your emotions. What you are feeling is a clue to what you need. If you have an emotional need, and you are meeting that need with food, you might want to seek a better way to meet your emotional needs. You might want to find something that meets your emotional needs BETTER than food does."

I got a hysterical phone call the next night. At first I could not even tell who it was. The woman on the line just kept yelling "Ten, ten, I only ate ten." Then I realized it was Lauren. She had tried the experience of savoring her M&Ms and really tasting them. On the eighth piece she tasted less flavor, but she could not believe it. On the ninth, it was really true. On the tenth M&M she was done. She was satisfied and she felt no compulsion to eat any more. At the next stoplight she folded the bag and put it in her glove compartment. For the last several years she has been eating ten M&Ms each night after work. (Oh, I must tell you that everything did not really turn out with a storybook ending as I have described so far. Lauren tried this exercise of savoring her M&Ms for the first time in March. She stored the bag of candy in her glove compartment. That is, until the first sunny warm day of spring when the candy melted and she discovered how unpleasant chocolate-covered papers and sunglasses really are. Now she keeps her M&Ms in her briefcase.)

******

Why does the concept of "savor your food" have such a profound effect on the way people eat? I'm sure there are many reasons. I will comment on the two significant reasons that stand out in my mind. First, let's look at the need to rebel against external controls.

Most people who work on changing their eating habits for weight loss or for medical reasons end up following some external plan, program, or recommendation from some expert. In the beginning, that seems to work for some people. In the beginning of a new eating program, some people seem to be able to drum up enough rational motivation to get started. However, if the person has started many, many eating programs in the past, they may not even be able to drum up enough rational motivation to last through the first day. Whenever it is, whether at the end of the first year or the first day, many people just can't take it anymore. Many people rebel against programs that they have to follow. It is like a two-year-old inside screams NO! Often this rebellion results in a binge. Sometimes the need to rebel against that program or authority is a whisper and a loss of motivation. In either case, there is a real need to rebel against an authority or program that dictates what should or should not be eaten.

The concept of "savoring your food" does NOT impose any external control on what you eat. There is nothing to rebel against. When you savor your food and notice the pleasure of eating and the pleasure of finding comfortable fullness, you are in charge of your eating. There is no need to rebel because there is no program or expert controlling your choices. You are making all your own choices. The two-year-old inside of you AND the intellectual side of you can both be happy.

The second reason that "savor your food" works so well has to do with the reasons people use food. If you are using food as fuel because you are hungry, it is very comfortable to savor your food and decide when you are full. What about those who use food for other reasons? Many people use food for emotional reasons. Actually, many people use food to tune out and disconnect from their emotions. Here is where the concept of "savor your food" has real power. Using this concept, you will be using the experience of eating TO TUNE IN to your emotional needs, instead of tuning out. When the next bite is not as delicious as the last, ask yourself, "Why eat it?" If you are eating for emotional reasons, you will get an emotional answer to this question. You may hear yourself saying, "I deserve it because I had a long day" or "because I can't stand feeling this way". If you hear yourself answer in a yelling tone of voice, it is a good guess that you are angry. You can use the experience of eating as a tool to tune in. Tuning-in is the key to meeting your emotional needs without using food as much.

What's Next After Savoring?

So, you have tried savoring your food. You have experienced tastes more, and you may have noticed your reactions or feelings more. You will continue to develop the skill of savoring your food from now on. But, savoring is just the doorway into a world of self-discovery. Savoring leads us to the next step. Remember asking yourself, "If this bite does not taste as good as the last, WHY EAT IT?" That is a good question! Let's focus on that for a while. *What do you need when you eat?*

Sometimes you just need food energy because you will not get to eat again for many hours. Sometimes you are compelled to eat by neurotransmitters released from the brain. Neuropeptide Y causes you to crave carbohydrates. Or it may be that galanin causes a craving for fats. Sometimes there are emotional reasons to eat. You may need a reward, comfort, distraction, etc. There can be many emotional reasons to eat.

First, let's consider emotional eating. When you notice the reasons you eat, you can develop more effective ways to meet those needs. This improves the quality of your life, not just your nutrition. There are two times when it is most useful to notice how you feel and what you need: BEFORE you eat, and AFTER you eat.

I encourage you to notice what you need BEFORE you eat. Too often we are in the habit of thinking of what *kind* of food we need. "Do I want something salty or sweet?" We are often accustomed to wrestling with the question: "To eat or not to eat?" No, that is *not* the question. When you focus on eating or not eating, you may divert yourself away from some more important, more real question. I am asking you to notice how you *feel* before you eat. Notice if there are any other *emotions* going on. I am asking you to increase your awareness. This is not easy. You will not do this all the time. Actually, you will only be able to use this increased awareness occasionally. Occasionally is fine! If you start to notice how you feel once in a while, you will be much closer to understanding yourself and what you need.

Once you are more aware of what you need, you can try other ways of meeting those needs. This sounds simple. It is not. You will go through a multi-step process to learn to meet your emotional needs without always using food. Right now, in the beginning, I am asking you to take note of your feeling and needs and write them down. You can use Your Own Book, the Don't Weight Workbook, or any paper you have around the house. You may choose to write down how you feel or what you need before you eat. Or, you may choose to do something else.

You may choose to tune in to your needs and feelings AFTER you eat. Sometimes, with the pressure of the decision over with, you can reflect on your emotions and discover what you needed when you ate. What if, when you are done eating, you have not gotten what you needed? You may be able to discover that need now, if you pay attention to it after you have eaten. What if eating really affected you? You can get an idea of what kind of effect you were looking for. This is vital information. When you know what you need, you may be able to come up with something more effective than food to meet those needs!

Did you notice that I put no importance on whether you ate or not? **The issue is not eating. The issue is building a life that meets your needs.** If you turn to food as a primary way to meet your needs, your needs will not get met. Food does not work well enough to meet emotional needs. If you take action and DO something that affects the quality of your life, more of your needs will be met. You will feel better and your life will be better too.

Emily

Emily found herself munching all the time. Her life was very hectic. She took care of the house, tended her husband who was ill, was matriarch of the family, and coped with her own disability. Now, it was time to prepare for the holidays.

There was so much to do. It was both overwhelming and stressful.

Munching helped. It really did help Emily feel better momentarily. When she ate sweets, she got comfort and pleasure. Her stress, however, seemed to keep building. Her injured leg really seemed to get worse as her weight increased. Now she had the worry of weight gain from excessive munching to add to her other stresses.

What could she do to cope with stress and feel better? Emily decided to start preparing for the holidays earlier than ever this year. That gave her less time pressure. She did a little each day. That gave her a feeling of effectiveness. She could see the progress. One of the most stressful experiences we can have is to feel powerless. Emily felt empowered when she accomplished her task each day. When she needed relief from stress, she would find one *small* task to do, and then really appreciate herself when it was done. This helped her to feel better than munching could have. This was a stress-relieving strategy she could use often. The question was not whether to munch or not. The question was how to feel better and fix her life. She started by identifying her feeling of stress.

Lists for Life

When you start to tune in to how you feel and what you need when you eat, you will discover many types of needs. I have already mentioned some of the most common needs that people often discover: comfort, reward, distraction, coping with anger, decompressing at the end of the day, coping with stress, etc. Once you have come to understand WHAT you need, how do you begin to meet those needs without always using food? What can you do?

Once again, you may find it useful to write. Writing is helpful because it is a way of making our thoughts and feelings tangible. Writing helps to take away the stress of trying to remember things. You don't have to review the list in your head, it is written down. You can relax and refer to your writing when you need to remember.

For example, think of a time when you had to buy a gift for someone and found yourself wandering around the department store looking for something to buy. Even if it were someone you knew very well, under the pressure of having to think of a gift right on the spot, it could be difficult to come up with anything appropriate. Often you would end up just buying something, anything that would get the job done, even if it was not quite the right gift for this person.

Now, imagine that you had been keeping a list. As you went through your daily life, whenever you saw something that would be the right gift for a friend or family member, you just added that gift idea to your list. You would gradually develop a list that you could refer to whenever you needed to buy a gift for someone. The gifts you gave your friends and family would be just the right gift and you would have reduced the stress of wandering aimlessly in the department store. You can use this same principal in your life to meet your own needs. You can make your own "Lists for Life".

Let's look at the moment when you got home from work. As you tuned in to your feelings, you noticed that you really needed to decompress from your workday. In the past, you have decompressed by eating. This worked. You wound down and calmed down. However, you often ate foods that had little or no nutrition. You end up overstuffed or groggy or just taking away your appetite for a nutritious dinner. This was a problem. This decompression munching is not really helping your life or your health. What else could you have done? At the moment when you walked in the door, you probably would not have been able to think of any other choices. After all, you needed to decompress, not to think. This was one of those times when you could have used a suggestion. Where could you get a suggestion for decompression activities that would really work for you? You get it <u>from yourself</u>!

Take a piece of paper. Write the word "Decompression" at the top. Divide the paper into four sections. Write one of these time intervals in each of the four sections:

1.) Just a few minutes
2.) About 15 minutes
3.) About half an hour
4.) An hour or more

Now you have a framework and all you need to do is use it. As you go through your life, keep your mind open for things that you can do that would help you decompress. Be patient with yourself. Over time ideas will come to you. You will not think of ideas all at once. You especially will not think of them at the time that you need to decompress. So, as you live your daily life, when you think of something that would help you decompress and relax, write down your idea in the section of your paper that most represents how long it would take to do that activity. Here are some ideas for decompressing that my clients have shared with me:

(Just a few minutes)

- Remove all the elastic from your body. In the summer, powder to cool-down. In the winter, lotion your skin to refresh. Then dress in cozy stay-at-home clothes.
- Since dehydration makes people feel tired, get a drink of water or non-caffeine tea (iced or hot.)
- Tell family or roommates that you need a few minutes ALONE, and **mean what you say**.
- Pet your cat.
- Pinch flowers in your garden.

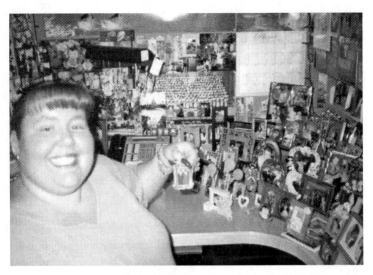

Meet your needs with hobbies, friends, and enjoyable activities in your life.

(About 15 minutes)

- Move through time and space, for your own pleasure, at your own pace. Take a gentle walk, in comfy shoes, just around your block or your yard. Breathe. Swing your arms. Feel the tension fall away like dust falls to the ground.
- Read your favorite self-esteem boosting magazine like Radiance, BBW, or Mode.
- Call a friend and talk about something that will help you feel better. You may want to vent about your day. You may not want to mention your day. Notice what would feel best to you.

You probably would not be able to think of all these things at the moment that you needed to decompress. However, you could look at a paper where all these ideas are already written down and CHOOSE which activity you will try today. You can make these same "Lists for Life" to use when you have "about a half hour" or "an hour or more" to spend on meeting your needs. Then you can look to these lists for ideas of alternate ways to meet your needs. You will find an activity that takes the amount of time you have available.

All you need to do is start to make your lists. Notice what you need: comfort, reward, distraction, or whatever. Keep your mind and heart open. When you discover what your needs are, make a list for each need. Put a word that represents your need at the top of each piece of paper where you will write your "Lists for Life". Notice how things affect you as you go through your days. Notice what meets your needs. As you find an activity that helps you calm down, decompress, feel comfort, vent anger, cheer up, (or whatever other needs you have), add that activity to your lists. You do not have to hold all these ideas in your head. You have them at your fingertips whenever you need them. When you use these lists you will meet your needs more effectively and you will feel more relaxed because you have so many constructive options from which to choose.

"The Food Cocoon"

There is a specific need that deserves specific attention. Sometimes, to meet this need, we use food. I don't mean just eating food, I mean wrapping yourself up in a food experience to insulate yourself from the world, or your family, or your problems, or something else. I call this the "food cocoon". To demonstrate this concept, I will tell a story from Carol's life:

Carol

Now in her early fifties, Carol is really making some changes. However, for DECADES she had been the main support for her very needy family. She had been the dependable one at work and often she was overloaded with responsibilities. Now, she is changing all that. No, it is not changing rapidly, but rather, it is changing gradually and comfortably, a little at a time.

Carol has added herself to the list of people who deserve her care and tending. Now, when there is a conflict of needs, she is likely to pay attention to what she needs as well as to what the other person needs.

Sometimes Carol feels on top of the world. It is so cool to watch this process. But, this is a process and as such, there are ups and downs. There are also times when Carol goes back to familiar exhausting patterns. Sometimes she is completely worn out. That is the time that I want to talk about here, the time when Carol can barely drag herself in the door at the end of an exhausting week.

On Fridays, Carol would gather up snacks and treats of food to take into her bedroom to watch TV. Her usually demanding and intrusive family had learned to leave her alone when she was in this kind of mood. At this one time, she was tired enough to let it all go. She used the food as an anesthetic. The food and TV would numb her mind and her feelings. She was in her "food cocoon". Nobody would bother her. No thoughts could survive the numbing neurotransmitters and the brain-sucking TV. She needed relief, and she got it.

The problem is that this relief had a very high price. The next morning, Carol felt as if she had a hangover. She had intestinal distress and even migraines at times. She felt awful about eating all that food that had no nutritional value, lots of unhealthy fats, and more food energy than her body ever needed. This was temporary relief and long-term misery. The food cocoon did not really work. The "food cocoon" was an illusion.

However, there was something REAL here. **Carol's need for relief was real.** That need was worth her attention. If she ignored her basic need for relief and just tried to use willpower to control her Friday night binges, she would be doomed to a wrestling match that would go on forever.

When she paid attention to her need for relief, then she could work this out.

Are there other ways to get relief? One thing that came to my mind was the idea that Carol said, *"my family knew better than to bother me when I was in this mood"*. Was her "food cocoon" the only time when Carol set firm boundaries and really let her family know that they MUST give her time and space to be alone? Could Carol get some relief by setting better boundaries with her family? As it turned out, that is exactly what did happen. Carol gave herself permission to chill out, have time alone, and enjoy her "constructive cocoon". Her belief that she had the right to this time alone helped her to be clear with her family and demand her own private time.

Once Carol had Friday evenings to herself (without the need to be anesthetized) there were other options available. Carol could do anything she wanted in her "constructive cocoon". What did she want? At the time that this manuscript is being written, Carol was in the middle of figuring that out. To begin with, she went back to her creative writing, began making special homemade papers with unique fibers and fragrances, and assembled artful bound books. Yes, she could do anything she wanted. And what a nice problem to have, tuning in and figuring out what she wants! It will be a blast to see what Carol comes up with next!

******

Think about your own life.
- Do you use your own "food cocoon" as a refuge?
- What needs of yours does your "food cocoon" meet?
- What are some other ways you can meet those needs?

This is a much more constructive way to look at the "food cocoon". Don't try to control it. Put your energy into building a constructive cocoon that really does meet your needs!

This is a delightful problem to have!
Instead of focusing on how to control your food binges,
now you have the challenge of figuring out
what you really want, what you really need,
and how to give it to yourself.

Do you, like Carol, need to give yourself explicit permission to take time for yourself? When you give yourself explicit permission, your inner self will not need to steal away into a "food cocoon" as the only way to get away from obligations.

Or maybe you are not overextended. Maybe you have been stagnant and just can't get yourself to DO anything. It is almost like inertia has you stuck and you can't get out. You may be using your "food cocoon" as solace from the pain of your depression. When you just can't do anything, eating is at least an activity to break the boredom, without getting you into a real activity. It may help to think of an **enjoyable**, small, (really small), activity to do. The activity you think of must be enjoyable in order for you to find the motivation to do it. Also, it must be small, even tiny. Sometimes tiny steps are the only steps you are able to take. Value tiny steps. They matter. You matter.

Figure out what you really want,
what you really need,
and give it to yourself.

Hand & Foot Massage
(A Physical Representation of Self-Care)

Remember when you discovered that you use food to meet many of your emotional needs? If you were not going to use food, you would need other ways to meet your emotional needs. Here are a few ideas. I did not think of this myself. A very clever client thought of this in one of our counseling sessions. I have, however, used it ever since. I use it myself. I recommend it to my other clients. You can use this whenever you need to relax, unwind, feel tended, feel nurtured, be appreciated, be acknowledged, center yourself, tune in to your physical self, and more. What could accomplish so many things?

An experience ...
An experience in pleasure ...
An experience you give yourself ...
A hand massage.

I know. This sounds silly. It is not. It is significant. When your right hand massages and tends your left hand, *you are experiencing a physical representation of this entire process of self-care.* You are not waiting around for someone else to give care. You are not distracting yourself from the pain of needing care. You are not being angry at your unmet needs. You are taking care of you. Every time you take care of you and tend yourself, you heal from the times in your life when you did not receive the care you needed. Every time you take care of yourself, the world becomes a safer place in which to live. You are building a sense of trust in yourself. You are learning to trust that YOU will take care of yourself and get your needs met. Take a moment. Take your left hand in your right. Give your left hand a wonderful massage. (Yes, you will give your right hand the same pampering next.)

Choices, choices, you have so many choices. Do you want a quick few second massage sitting right there at your desk? Will you simply squeeze and press wherever it feels good on the palm, on the fingers, at the tips? You don't even need hand lotion for this kind of massage. When one hand is done, roll your shoulders, sit up tall, lay your hands on a pillow on your lap or just on your desk, and do the other hand. Breathe. Be.

Or, do you want to sit down, when tasks are set aside for a while, and pamper yourself? This is a time when you might take a little longer and use hand cream or lotion. When your hands are slippery, you will find all sorts of motions that feel good. Rubbing in little circles, sliding your fingers or knuckles across the palm, pulling as you slip down the finger to a little press on the finger pad. Ahhh ... you deserve this. And you deserve twice as much relaxation and enjoyment because you have an entire other hand to go. Change sides and let the other hand feel tended.

There is more than just relaxation going on here. When one hand is being massaged and relaxing, the other hand is getting a gentle, rhythmic, vigorous, workout. The muscles, tendons, and ligaments in your working hand are all being used as you squeeze, press, and kneed the left hand. This is great exercise. My clients with arthritis and carpal tunnel have found that their symptoms actually reduce when they use this massage technique a few times a day!

Oh, but there is more. A healing art called reflexology has been used for centuries. According to reflexology, there are points and regions on the hands and feet that correspond to areas of the body and organs. My clients report that they find themselves pressing on or massaging specific areas of their hand or foot, just naturally, with not specific intent. Often, when we look at a reflexology chart, we see that the specific spot in the hand or foot that they were drawn to press or massage is precisely the spot that corresponds to a body area or organ where they have had illness or problems. This is not scientific evidence. This is simply an interesting anecdotal report. However, since I find no negative side effects to gentle hand massage, I think it is interesting to entertain the possibility of other positive benefits.

I mention the hand massage first because most people who have two hands can do this exercise. (I have clients with only one hand who accomplish similar results pressing their one hand on and against a wooden or plastic ball or rounded surface.) The next type of massage may require some creativity for some people to implement. Let's explore the foot massage. First, I will comment on massage for those who can reach their feet. I recommend that you sit in bed with support for your back. Sometimes it is best with a pillow tucked under your butt so that you can lean forward more comfortably. Many people find it easier to move one foot within reach while the other foot hangs off the side of the bed. Some people are comfortable with both feet within reach. One position is NOT better than the other. The best position is the one that works for you and is comfortable (especially on your back.) So, there you are, sitting, back supported, and comfortable. Now you can enjoy your foot massage. You will find that you can press and squeeze harder on the foot than on the hand. You may want to use your knuckles to get the right pressure on your foot while still being gentle on your fingers. Since your feet are used to carrying your weight, it may feel good to actually pound gently on your heels. Your toes however are more delicate. You may like to pull gently and press on the pads, just like on the fingers.

What if you cannot reach your feet? What if your hands are quite far from them indeed? Here is where another clever client has helped us all out. (There probably are fancy tools in specialty health catalogues for this purpose, but I find this client's idea works great.) Get a wooden spoon. You can choose a short or long handled spoon, depending on how far you need it to reach. The weight, smooth texture, and shape of a simple wooden spoon makes the perfect tool for tapping, pressing, and massaging your feet if you cannot reach. You can use the rounded tip of the spoon to press with specific pressure in one spot. You can softly tap your arch with the flattened round bottom of the spoon. When firmer pounding would feel good on your heel, you can use the edge of the spoon. Once you have gently relaxed and stimulated your feet with tapping, pressing, and gentle pounding, you can use the same spoon to apply cream to your feet. Put a dab of cream on the back of the spoon and apply with gentle circles. The side of the spoon will slip, sometimes with a giggle, between your toes. Enjoy. You and your feet deserve it.

Oh, but there is more. While you are giving yourself a nice foot massage in whatever fashion works for you and your body, you are also doing something else very important. You are stretching your low back, upper back, hamstrings, and inner thighs. Since you are massaging both feet, you are getting an even symmetrical stretch on both sides of your body. Feel it. Breathe into the stretch as you reach for your foot. Easy, easy, only stretch as much as is comfortable.

What is happening to your upper back, shoulders, arms, and hands while you are giving yourself a foot massage? They are all working and using the muscles of your upper body. Make sure that you alternate hands and use your right **and** left hands when you work on your feet. This will help you to work the muscles on both sides of your upper body. You can increase the strength and stamina of your shoulders, arms, and hands just by enjoying more frequent foot massages. It is kind of nice how everything is connected.

The Tea Ritual

I know eastern cultures have had tea rituals for centuries. When I think of human nature and the components of a tea ritual, I think all people can benefit from the aroma, relaxation, and structure of the tea ritual. I was not the one to bring this great idea into my life. Oh, I drank tea. But, that is not the same as a tea ritual. My clients were the ones to instruct me in the true value of this activity. When one client had an idea to drink tea to relax, I told other clients about it. As other clients used this idea, each one added another way that they could benefit from drinking, preparing, and serving tea. Eventually a ritual evolved. I encourage you to try this idea and develop your own individual ritual that meets your specific needs. But, first there is some background information you will find useful.

I must start with some information about the human brain. Our olfactory center, the part of the brain that processes our sense of smell, is *very* deep in the brain. This was one of the first parts to develop in the evolution of the human brain. Therefore our sense of smell is our most basic sense. Smells and aromas profoundly affect us. Our *emotions* and our moods are affected by what we smell. We can use this fact when we seek ways to meet our emotional needs.

Next, I want to comment on breathing. Deep breathing relaxes and reduces stress. We all know it. We just don't do it enough. Try it right now. Lift your ribcage so you have room to breathe. Look up from this book. Slowly inhale through your nose as you feel the cool air fill your lungs. Slowly exhale through your mouth and hear your sigh of relaxation. Anytime you participate in an activity that encourages deep slow breathing, you are encouraging relaxation. This is worth remembering since relaxation and stress reduction are primary human needs.

The last concept that I want to mention is the effect that habits have on our emotions. People are creatures of habit. When we do something the first time we must think about it quite a lot. After we have done an activity many times, we get in a habit and we do not have to think as much about our actions. Our emotions are also involved. Habitual actions, or rituals, tend to evoke the same habitual emotional response time after time. We get used to doing an action and feeling the corresponding emotion. It is all part of the habit. Some habits trigger anxiety and tension. Some habits trigger comfort and familiarity.

**It takes just as long to form a constructive habit
as it does to form a destructive habit.**

**We can choose to foster habits that improve our lives.
Part of the process of building a healthy lifestyle
is to gradually add constructive habits that
are comfortable and self-perpetuating.**

How can we use human reactions to aroma, the relaxation of deep breathing, and the comfort/familiarity of habits to meet our emotional needs? My answer is the "Tea Ritual". I will not tell you what the ritual should be. Instead I will ask you a series of questions that will assist you in developing your own ritual.

- How will you make your tea? It is up to you. Some people like the speed of the microwave. Some people like the peaceful sound of boiling water on the stove. Experiment. Choose what you want.
- What cup feels good to you? Do you want a sturdy mug or a dainty china cup? You may like different cups for different tea or moods.
- Where will you sit when you drink your tea? What kind of chair will feel most comfortable while still supporting good posture? You need good posture in order to breathe deeply.
- What do you want to look at while you sip your tea? This is very important. Select a spot where you will be looking at something pleasant. Would you like to look out a window at a tree in the breeze? Do you want to watch your fish in the aquarium? I suggest you do NOT watch television. TV often has an anesthetic effect that causes tired tension rather than relaxation.
- What sounds do you want to listen to while you drink your tea? Do you want to listen to music, the breeze in the trees, or a wind chime? Think about it and set yourself up to hear pleasant sounds.
- What kind of tea do you like? I suggest you try non-caffeine or decaffeinated tea in any flavor you want. Some teas claim to have qualities like "calming" or "relaxing" or "refreshing". Please consider these claims to be possibilities and *trust your own reactions* to choose what you like best.
- What do you want to put in your tea? If you can learn to enjoy tea plain, that is better. Your tea ritual will be more

useful if it does not stimulate your appetite. If you like sweets, try the smallest amount of sugar or honey that satisfies you.

When you have experimented and answered these questions for yourself, you will have a ritual that you can use repeatedly. As you make your tea, breathe and relax. Think calming thoughts. If unpleasant thoughts intrude, you may select a helpful positive phrase to repeat in your mind. You cannot think two thoughts at the same time. Keep your positive thoughts flowing. It will become a habit.

As you brew and sip your tea, inhale the aroma. Breathe. Feel the scent fill you. Picture the rehabilitating oxygen flow into your lungs. Breathe. Exhale the used air, making room for more delightful aroma. Relax. After you get in this relaxing habit, all you will need to do is imagine the aroma and breathe deeply. Relaxation will descend on you like a soft rain. Once you are practiced, you can give this to yourself anytime you want. (I used to carry my favorite tea bag in my purse so that I could inhale the scent when I needed to relax. Later I used the memory of that lovely scent to help me relax.)

You can enjoy long tea rituals or tiny brief ones. In hot weather, you can enjoy the aroma of the tea brewing and then pour it over ice for a cool drink. You can do what you choose. You have one more tool to use when you need relaxation, comfort, calm, and much more. You deserve to feel good.

Have You Eaten Enough Today?

After years and years of being told that you are overweight because you eat too much, did you ever think somebody would tell you to eat more? Well, it is happening today. I am telling you that to build your healthy eating style, you may need to eat more. During this process, we will focus on what you *should* eat, instead of what you should not eat.

There is NO RESTRICTED eating in this process. You are encouraged to eat foods that are good for your health, (you won't hear me telling you to avoid or restrict any particular foods.) You are encouraged to be more aware of when you are satisfied, not to limit portions.

**It takes
every minute of
every hour of
every day to
NOT eat something.**

**It takes just a moment
to eat something healthy.**

When you focus on selecting and eating all the wonderful tasty foods that are good for you, your time and energy will be spent eating healthy foods and enjoying every bite. This healthy eating is a task that can take up all the energy you used to put into restricting and limiting your eating.

Many people "get the munchies" in the evening. If you are one of those people, ask yourself: "Have I eaten enough today?" "Did I eat enough fruit and veggies?" "Did I eat when I was hungry?" "How was my nutrition?" If you realize that you didn't eat enough veggies, you could have a salad or bowl of vegetable soup. If you notice that you were low on protein today, you could have a high protein snack. If you realize that you were hungry during the day, had nothing to eat, and therefore stayed hungry too long, you could plan a way to avoid that situation in the future.

This is a fundamentally different look at healthy eating. There is NO portion control. There is NO deprivation. If you have an emotional need to put a lot of energy into this healthy eating process ... fine. Think a lot about these constructive concepts and focuses. Ask yourself the questions in the above paragraph often.

If you can't stand the thought of putting energy into thinking about your eating ... FINE. Ask yourself these constructive questions whenever seem to be worrying about food or body image issues anyway. You would not be spending any more energy. You would just be redirecting your already used energy into a more constructive focus.

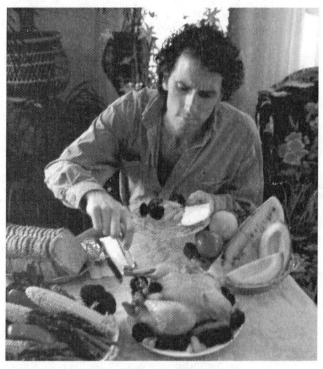

Everybody of every size, large or small, needs to eat enough foods for good nutrition.

The recommended number of servings of fruits and vegetables per day is FIVE. I call these foods the "live foods". Few people get enough live foods in the course of the day. If you want to improve your healthy eating, **eat more fruits and vegetables**. This sounds like a simple goal to achieve. **This is not a simple goal.** This goal, like so many lifestyle goals, is much more complicated than it seems at first glance. Be prepared to go through a process of trying things that sometimes work, and sometimes don't. Have you ever planned on eating more fruits and veggies, but somehow it just didn't work out? Welcome to the human race! Be patient with yourself. Consider it a mystery. Work on solving the mystery, taking one step at a time. Ask yourself questions like these:

- Do I have access to fruits and veggies? You may need to change the way you shop and store your produce. This could involve reworking your entire schedule to include a different shopping pattern. You may need to learn new ways of ordering food at restaurants or come up with better ways of packing your lunch.
- Do I have enjoyment-based motivation to eat my fruits and veggies? The most common reason I hear for not liking fruits and veggies is that they "feel like diet food". You may not be able to motivate yourself just because "it is good for you". You can motivate yourself with enjoyment, with foods that taste and look appetizing. Find delicious ways to enjoy these healthy foods, then you will eat them because you enjoy them. Keep a beautiful fruit bowl on your table or desk. Then you will eat fruit because it looks so tasty and it is so convenient.
- Are there any problems with eating fruits and veggies that I need to solve? Some people have digestive problems, mouth or tooth pain, gas, etc. That does not mean you need to give up on getting your healthy "live food". Get creative. Try fruits and veggies that are new to you. Experiment with food combinations and time of day that you eat. If you have gas, try Beano™ (a natural food enzyme that you eat with your food that helps digestion and reduces gas.) If you have mouth or tooth pain, see your dentist and solve the problem. In general, that's the idea: Don't just live with a problem that gets in the way of taking care of yourself, work on solving it!

This is part of the process of "back up, don't beat up". You will plan to eat better foods. Sometimes you will. Those are times to notice what helped you to take care of yourself. Sometimes you will not eat as you had planned. Those are the times to back up and think about what got in the way. Writing may be a useful tool as you think through these problems. It can help you respect how complicated the process of change is. Writing can help you appreciate the effort that you put into eating healthier. It is worth the effort to include more fruits and veggies in your day. In an experiment to explored the Dietary Approaches to Stop Hypertension (DASH), researchers showed that people can lower their blood pressure in only two weeks by eating more fruits and vegetables and less saturated fat!

If you feel like you really want to make a difference in the way you eat, pay attention to what you DO (rather than what you want to avoid.) Think about what foods you want to INCREASE. Don't think about limiting or eliminating foods. When you get the munchies, ask yourself:

"Have I eaten enough today?"

The munchies are not the problem.
The fact that you may need better nutrition
and more fruits and vegetables
might be the problem.

This can be a rather enjoyable problem to solve. Get some tasty and nutritious food and enjoy it. Whether you are eating for fuel or for entertainment, savor your food. When the next bite is not as delicious as the last, ask yourself: "Why eat it?" You can answer that question and do whatever you choose.

To Eat or Not to Eat, That is NOT the Question!

What if your nutrition has been fine? You did eat when you were hungry. You did eat healthy foods. But still, you find yourself in a wild search for "something". You find yourself obsessed with the question: "Do I want salt or sweet?" You want to eat. You feel driven to eat something. But, you know you're not really hungry. You know you ate your nutritious foods today. The old restrictive eating thoughts creep in. "I really *should* not eat any more." You descend into a war of willpower over cravings. You get caught up in the next question: "To eat, or not to eat?" It feels like that is the central conflict of your evening. Heck, when it is happening it feels like the central conflict of your LIFE. **What is going on here?**

Now, that is a good question! What is going on here? THAT is the question. How do you find the answer? It is different for everybody. It is different for the same person at various times. You need some tools to help you answer this question. When you are in the middle of a food craving, what is going on? When you're not hungry, and you're already nourished with food, there must be some other reason you are embroiled in the question: "to eat, or not to eat?" Focusing on that question may be your learned coping skill. It is a familiar, and ineffective, way to cope. You need some other ways to discover and cope with the real issue.

Possible Tools (use the ones that seem right for you):

- **Talk to somebody.** Even if it is yourself, talk to somebody. Out loud. It is important that you talk out loud so that you will finish your sentences. You see, when we think things through, we tend to jump from thought to thought without coming to the end of each thought. It is as if we assume we know the end of the thought and there is no need to finish it. When you talk out loud and hear what you have to say, you may be surprised at the end of your sentences. You may find some emotional drama going on inside of you. You may find some reasons for how you feel and what you do. Then you can take action to address what is really going on. (It is probably not about the food at all.)

ET

Yes, I do mean ET, the little alien in the movie. ET saved Nancy's life. She was in an unbearable situation. She had no way out. She had no one to talk to. There was no friend who could possibly understand, no family available, no access to a therapist. Nancy was in a deep situational depression and she could not get out of the situation. A poster of ET was on her wall. She talked to him. She told him stories, feelings, ideas. He was there for her. She used these verbalizations to keep her head above water. She did not acknowledge to herself that she was feeling suicidal. She just wanted to be gone, to disappear. But she did not make plans to act on those thoughts. I truly believe that talking to ET was a major reason she held on until the situation did change.

Nancy eventually came to understand the situations in her life that caused the depression. Now, she knows herself amazingly well. She still gets depressed sometimes. I suspect she still talks to ET. And she keeps solving problems, one by one, so that she can build a life without unbearable situations. She is building a life that meets her needs.

- **Write.** Sit in a peaceful place, get out your paper and pen, and just ramble. I suggest bulleted phrases. You can get your thoughts out fast and furiously. Let 'em roll out of your head and onto the paper. Don't scrutinize. Don't assess. Just ramble. This type of free association may lead you to some amazing awareness of your emotions or thoughts that could surprise you. It may lead you to some reason you are standing in front of the pantry concentrating on food. It probably will have little to do with food.

- **Try "just colors".** If you don't like talking, and you don't like writing, you still need a tool to understand yourself. Often, I have worked with clients who feel uncomfortable with both talking and writing. I learned this technique from an ingenious woman who was seeking a way to express herself without talking or writing. She kept a notebook. It was not filled with paragraphs or bulleted points. Instead it was filled with art paper (the kind that holds up to water color paints.) She did write a brief topic line at the top of each page: "Friday, when I got home from parent-teacher night", "Saturday evening, early", "after gardening", etc. Then on the page were just colors. Whatever colors (or no colors, she often painted shades of gray) she wanted to paint. The colors swirled in wet melted puddles, or jabbed in jagged dry strokes, or dotted in crowds or alone. It was amazing. This notebook was a tool for understanding what she could not say or write. It was a tool for understanding herself. We did end up talking about the feelings, events, and ideas expressed on the pages. But it was just colors that opened the door. You can open the door to your understanding any way that you want. You deserve to be understood and tended, especially by you.

> **When it seems like the question is:**
> **"to eat, or not to eat",**
> **take a moment to ask a different question.**
> **Ask: "What's going on here?"**

Give yourself some time and use whatever tools work for you. Peek inside of yourself. Try to understand how you are feeling right now. Can you tell what triggered this feeling? How can you cope with that trigger? What do you need?

There are lots of questions. These questions are so much more effective than the old question about eating. Ask yourself questions that will help you fix your life. Do what you can to solve the problems that those questions uncover. **Try to focus on your life, not your food.** What about those times when, even after you have tended your emotions, you still want to eat?

First, Eat Something Healthy

You're hungry, or
you have the "munchies", or
you just want "something", or
you have a craving.
You want to eat.

You have paid attention to what you need emotionally. When it seemed like you needed comfort, you already did comfort yourself in non-food ways. When you needed relief from boredom, you did something interesting. When you needed to tune-out, you actually did tune in to the issue at hand, even if it was just a little bit. And, even after paying attention to your emotional needs:

You're still hungry, or
you still have the "munchies", or
you still just want "something", or
you still have a craving.
You still want to eat.
Now, what do you do?

If tuning in to your emotional needs did not give you the information necessary to take care of yourself, maybe you can get more information if you take away the question of "to eat or not to eat" all together. Next, try something with which you are more familiar. Eat. Whenever you are actually stomach-growling hungry (even if your mind tells you that you should not be hungry), EAT. Only, I suggest that you eat something healthy. I recommend that you HAVE A HEALTHY FOOD CHOICE AVAILABLE TO YOU AT ALL TIMES. If you were taking care of a little one for the day, you would always have healthy snacks stuffed in your bag, just in case the little one got hungry. Give yourself the same care.

When you are not actually stomach-growling hungry, but you really want something anyway; it is all right to EAT. Just eat something healthy first. Think about your day, ask yourself: "Have I eaten enough fruits and veggies?" "Have I eaten enough protein?" "Have I had enough water?" Think about the nutritious foods you still need today, and give yourself the food your body needs.

After you have eaten something healthy, give your body and mind some time to react. (It takes twenty minutes for food you have eaten to affect the glucose levels in your blood so that your brain gets the chemical signal that you are full.) Then, when a little time has gone by, you will notice that your craving is gone or your craving is still tugging at you.

If your craving is gone after eating something healthy, move on with your day or your evening.

If your craving is still tugging at you, EAT WHATEVER YOU WANT.

Yes, that is what I said, eat whatever you want. There is only one catch. It is very important that you REALLY ENJOY WHAT YOU EAT.

Savor every bite.

Especially since you are eating to satisfy a craving, this is the time to savor your food and NOTICE WHEN YOU ARE SATISFIED. When you are satisfied, why eat anymore? This is a comfortable time to stop eating. There is no wrestling match with your willpower, no restriction. You just ate some healthy foods and some "entertainment" food. That's fine.

I want you to imagine this scenario:

- You had a craving and you tuned in to your emotional needs. When you discovered "What was going on here?", you addressed your emotional need. Sometimes, at that point, the craving went away. You would be finished dealing with your craving. But sometimes the craving persists. Fine. Cope with it instead of fighting it.
- You continued to crave and you ate something healthy first. Sometimes, eating the healthy food ends the craving. You are done. Sometimes the craving persists. Fine. Cope with it instead of fighting it.
- You still crave and you ate what you craved. This time, instead of eating guiltily in the closet, slipping the food past your awareness and your taste buds, this time you tasted and savored every bite. You were present and aware. You can do what you CHOOSE, instead of what you are compelled to do.
- You enjoyed what you ate, and stopped when you were satisfied. No big deal. It is just some food. You enjoyed it. And you are comfortably full without overeating. No willpower required.

Can you imagine it? How would you feel? Isn't this much better than an uncontrolled guilt filled "binge"? Would you end up eating more healthy foods and less entertainment foods when you cope with cravings this way? Would you feel less guilt? Can you see that there is NO DEPRIVATION in this way of coping with cravings?

There is no restriction imposed. When you cope with cravings by meeting your emotional needs and then eating something healthy first, you are tuning in to what you need. You are taking care of yourself instead of forcing yourself to use willpower and stay "on a program". Because you are internally motivated and you are not on a program, you cannot go "off the program". If you try to cope with cravings this new way, and you don't do as you intended ... that's all right. You are in the middle of learning this new way of coping. There will be another craving. You will get another chance to practice this new way of coping with your next craving.

Cravings can be scary. Especially if you have felt wildly out of control with your eating in the past. Practice this new way of coping. Let some time pass. Gradually, you will be less scared. When your next craving hits you, take a breath, tune in, and take care of yourself. You deserve it.

Your Appetite Can be an ASSET

I used to travel with my husband on business trips. I functioned as the hostess for wives who were also on the trip. We called these trips "vacations". Indeed we traveled to Hawaii, Spain, and resorts all over the country. I had the unique experience of traveling both when I was a compulsive eater and when I had made peace with food.

Traveling as a compulsive eater was an interesting experience. There was food everywhere. And there was permission to eat. After all, this was vacation. At breakfast there was a display of pastries, and I could have all that I wanted. I wanted a lot. Mid-morning we were stopping at a little shop for candies. And it was perfectly acceptable to have candy on vacation. After all, I would go back to dieting when I returned. This went on all day and all night, eating every two or three hours. The first day I really enjoyed myself. The second day, the food had lost its wonder. By the third day, I felt kind of sick. But I was on vacation. How could I turn down these delicious treats that I would never have again? The vacation became a roller coaster ride of eating and nausea. I still enjoyed the eating, briefly. I spent most of the vacation waiting for that sick feeling to go away … so I could eat again.

Traveling only a few years later, when I had made peace with food, was a completely different experience. I wanted to enjoy what I ate and how I felt <u>after</u> I ate. I learned from experience that a good breakfast helped me feel better all day. It was easy to choose a lower fat breakfast and fresh fruits. I also enjoyed some pastry. This time, when the next bite did not taste as delicious as the last, I choose to stop eating **so that I could enjoy myself more**. I was seeking that delightful balance between eating for pleasure and feeling comfortable afterward. Mid-morning, when we were at the shops full of candies or treats, I had two questions to ask myself: Do I want to be hungry for lunch so that I can enjoy lunch more? Or do I want to enjoy some of this food now? I could answer yes to either question. I could answer yes to both questions. What I would not do was to eat until I felt sick. I was on vacation. I deserved to enjoy myself. I would not spoil my vacation by overeating to discomfort.

I remembered a saying I had learned in Spanish class:

"Hunger is the best seasoning."

(Unfortunately, I remember it only in English because we learned by translating everything.) When I was in the middle of compulsive eating and bulimia, I had not experienced hunger for years. When I recovered from my eating disorders, I paid attention to eating, enjoyment, and satisfaction. I learned that hunger was truly the best seasoning. Everything tasted better when I was hungry. So, when I was on vacation, getting hungry was a good thing. It meant that I would enjoy my next meal even more. I would eat healthy food at meals and enjoy tastes of desert. I would have bits of delicious snacks between meals so that I would not spoil my appetite. My appetite became something that I cultivated. I wanted to be hungry when it was time to eat. I paced my eating for maximum enjoyment. After all, I was on vacation.

This is a complete change from the familiar idea of "controlling your appetite". This is really different from the idea that your appetite is "the problem", or the feeling of being "at war with your appetite".

Your appetite can be an asset to healthy eating, not an enemy!

When your appetite is an asset that enhances enjoyment in eating, you have no need for control. You will eat comfortable amounts of food, because it is more pleasurable. You will find yourself saying "No, thank you" because you are looking forward to your next meal and you want to feel your appetite for the next meal. The only effort you need is the effort to keep your focus on truly enjoying yourself both now and later. The only willpower you need is the willpower to keep looking at the broader picture so that you can enjoy yourself both now and later. What a difference!

Eating at Home: A New Way to Look in the Pantry or Fridge

I want you to imagine our ancestors, the cave men. We all know that the ones who survived to procreate were the ones with tendencies and characteristics that helped them overcome the obstacles of the day. Starvation was one of the main obstacles. The cave man who tended to walk right by a juicy root or ripe berry with no need to eat it did not live long.

The cave man who responded to visual stimuli (who was motivated to eat whenever he saw food) lived longer and had more descendants. Human beings have inherited the tendency to respond when we see food. This drive comes from the most primitive part of our brain. Willpower cannot win out over millions of years of biology. We can, however, use our biology to help us eat healthy tasty foods in comfortable amounts.

When you are looking for something to eat, DO NOT LOOK IN THE PANTRY. When you are looking for something to eat, DO NOT LOOK IN THE REFRIGERATOR. If you do, you may be visually stimulated to eat whatever you see. What you see may not be what would be good for you. We have exposure to so much more food than the cave man. Our natural tendency to eat what we see can result in unbalanced nutrition. I have another idea for you to try. When you are looking for something to eat, look someplace where all the foods are good for you. Look someplace with variety and tasty foods. You will have to create this place for yourself. The good news is that it only takes a little of your time.

Get a piece of paper and write "Breakfast Menu" at the top. Now, think of an enjoyable nutritious breakfast. Start your menu with that breakfast. Keep thinking and add as many healthy, tasty, breakfast choices as you can. If you cannot think of choices right away, set the list on your counter and add breakfast choices over the next few weeks as you come up with ideas. What you will have is a customized, personalized, healthy, tasty, enjoyable menu of breakfast foods from which you can choose. When you need to decide what to eat for breakfast, *open your menu and choose anything you want*. Now, your inherited tendency to want what you see is an asset in your nutrition. What you see is good for you!

You can make your own delicious and nutritious menu for lunch, dinner, and snacks too. Some of my clients have added artwork or made their menus on computer. Use your visual senses to enhance your healthy eating choices. Use your own menus to *relax* and choose whatever you want from the foods you have listed on your menu. These foods are truly good for your body. AFTER you have decided what you want, then go and find the ingredients in your pantry or refrigerator. You can have variety, spontaneity, and healthy eating. Just decide what you want from your menu *first,* and then look in your pantry or refrigerator.

Eating at Restaurants: A New Way to Look at a Menu

Once more I want you to picture your cave man ancestor. Think about your inherited tendency to be influenced by the sight of food. You can understand why most restaurant menus now use photographs of delicious foods alongside the written description. What can you do to increase the chance you will choose a meal that is healthier for you? Look someplace where there are pictures of meals that are more healthy. Look in your own head.

When you sit down at a restaurant, do not look at the menu. Sit down, settle in, and think about what you want. From your own experience, from your own appetites, select what you want. Picture chicken, fish, vegetable lasagna, and more. Notice your reactions to each option and think about it. What sounds good to you? When you have found something in your own head that you feel like ordering, *now* you are ready to look in the menu. However, you are not looking to see what the menu may suggest to you. You are looking for a specific type of dish and where it may be located on the menu. You know what you want. You just need to complete the hunt by finding it on the menu. The "cave man" side of you is satisfied because you hunted through your own list of foods (in your head) and chose what appealed to you. The "modern man" side of you is satisfied because you get to enjoy the convenience of hunting through the menu and finding food that is good for you. What a treat to sit down, think of exactly what you want, and have it delivered to your table!

An Exercise in Halves

The most important part of this exercise is your motivation and the goal you set as you try the exercise. You may be tempted to turn this into an exercise to help you eat less food. That is normal. It is just not helpful. If your motivation and goal becomes controlling your portion size, then you would have turned this exercise into just another diet behavior. When done with the correct goal in mind, this exercise leads you to the OPPOSITE of dieting. This exercise is a tool for you to use as you journey away from external controls on your eating toward INTERNAL choices.

**The goal of this exercise is
for you to enjoy your food,
your health, and your life.**

Do you ever find yourself uncomfortably full at the end of a meal? Sometimes it is quite a surprise. While you were eating you were not uncomfortable. Then a few minutes after you finish ... boom ... that overstuffed feeling hits you. Wouldn't it be helpful to increase your awareness of how you feel *while* you are in the middle of your meal? That would allow you to make choices that were more comfortable. That would allow you to enjoy both your meal *and* a comfortable level of fullness afterward. Try this.

- At a meal of your choice, decide to try the "exercise in halves". This is a simple exercise, although it can have profound results and lead you to great personal insight.

- When you start your meal, divide it in half. If you have a sandwich, cut it in half. If you have a pile of mashed potatoes, just scoop one half slightly apart from the other half. You do not have to make a big production out of this. It only takes a moment and it can be done subtly.
- Next, enjoy and savor the first half of your meal. Experience it. Really taste it. When you are done with half of your meal, stop. Take a moment to notice how you feel. Notice your level of fullness. Notice if you are satisfied or if you would like to have more.
- If you are full and satisfied, why eat more? (That is why they invented plastic wrap and microwaves.) If you are not yet full, then you are ready for the next step in the "exercise in halves".
- With the food left on your plate, divide it in half. Enjoy and savor the next half of your meal. When you are done with this half, notice how you feel. Have you reached a comfortable level of fullness? If so, why eat any more? If not, divide the food left on your plate in half... You get the idea. Eat half and then focus on how you feel.

The goal of the "exercise in halves" is to eat as much of your meal as you want, as much as leaves you comfortable. When you experiment with this exercise, you are likely to be able to accomplish these two results:

1.) Thoroughly enjoying your meal while eating
2.) Achieving a comfortable level of fullness after eating

This "exercise in halves" is a tool to use if and only if it helps you in your individual process toward healthy eating. This exercise is designed to help you develop internal choices and increased awareness of how you feel and what you need. It is not a tool for portion control. If you use this exercise to trick yourself into eating less, you may find that you react the same way you would if you were dieting.

Use this exercise as long as you find it to be helpful. Don't use it if you find yourself having some uncomfortable reaction to it. (Although, you may find it valuable to think through your reaction, in case that is part of your individual process.) Remember that this is YOUR process. You are the only one in the entire world who will react the way you do. There are lots of tools, exercises, ways of thinking, etc. It is up to you to notice your reaction to trying any of the ideas presented here. It is up to you to use or not use anything that you choose. This is not a program where you are required to follow the steps. This is a process that you are designing for yourself.

You are leading yourself through your own individual process as you read this book and experience your reactions. Try the "exercise in halves" if you think it will be helpful. Try it at least once even if you don't. Skip this exercise altogether if you feel it will reduce your healthy eating or trigger a negative reaction. Trust yourself and keep thinking.

What about Water?

Human beings are supposed to drink water. It's that simple ... or is it? You make a resolution to drink more water and a few weeks later you have forgotten all about it. You feel stupid for not being able to do this one little thing. You ask yourself, "Why is it so difficult to do something as simple as drinking water?"

Because it is NOT simple. It is a complicated process to change your habits. There are several side effects of drinking water that need to be considered. Nobody ever talks about the difficulties. When you think of a task as simple, it seems like anybody could accomplish that task. However, when you acknowledge that a task is difficult, you can respect your efforts as you work toward success.

Let's consider what is necessary in order for you to hydrate yourself. You need to have access to water or other beverages without caffeine or too much sugar. Where do you spend your days? Do you have access to water at that location? Do you need to keep a water bottle near you? How will you carry your water bottle? Do you like cold water? How will you keep it cold? See, this is not simple, but it is a task that you can accomplish if you let yourself think the problem through.

There is another issue that is associated with drinking water that is often overlooked. When you drink water, you will have to go to the bathroom more often than when you dehydrate yourself. I have many clients who limit their water intake so that they won't have to interrupt their workday. Think about this for a moment. Do you ever see other workers taking a break because they just HAVE to have a cigarette? Yep. Well then, think of yourself as being addicted to healthy living and you just HAVE to stay hydrated and go to the bathroom more often. You have the right.

Actually, when you get away from your work for a bit and take a short walk, you may even help your overall concentration, alertness, and ability to function. Human beings are not designed to sit in one spot for long periods of time. Getting up and moving is good for your mind and for your body. You will be a better worker when you take care of yourself.

There is one time when you do not want to have to get up and go, that is nighttime. Most people find that if they drink more in the daytime and less in the evening, they will minimize having to get up at night to go to the bathroom. Reducing caffeine in the late afternoon and evening will also help with this goal. Play around with your water and your schedule.

Get creative about how you enjoy water. If you don't like plain water, don't drink it. Forcing yourself to drink something you don't like will feel like a dreadful chore and you will soon abandon the goal of drinking more water. Put a slice of citrus in your water. Try it filtered, brewed into teas without caffeine, with a splash of fruit juice, etc. Find a beverage that is good for you and tastes good so that you will continue for a lifetime to drink the water you need.

Healthy Lifestyles for All Sizes

Traditional dieting is often the <u>cause</u> of binge eating and compulsive eating. Think about a day when you decided to take control of your eating. You ate a small sensible breakfast and lunch. You passed right by the donuts at the office. You stayed strong and said no to cookies in the afternoon. But then, that evening, you found yourself eating everything you could get your hands on! Welcome to the human race. You were having a normal reaction to an abnormal situation of deprivation.

This cycle is repeated daily by millions of people who are trying to lose weight. Sometimes the time frame changes. Sometimes they "are good" for months at a time, particularly before a special event like a wedding or class reunion. They do lose weight. Then, in the weeks or months that follow they become part of the 90% or more of dieters who gain back all they have lost.

Those who think they are fat often internalize society's stereotypes and perceive themselves as lazy, gluttonous, unworthy, and unlovable. This can lead to desperation. When Fen-Phen was taken off the market, we saw many reports of people who wanted to take the drugs even though they were proven to be dangerous: "I would rather die than stay fat".

What can you do if you are worried about your weight? Do everything you can that is reasonable to build a healthy lifestyle. Seek out the support and education you need to develop these skills:

- Eat nutritious foods when you are hungry.
- Stop eating when you are satisfied.

- Meet your emotional needs without always using food.
- Enjoy exercise regularly.

**Work toward doing everything reasonable
to build your healthy lifestyle ... relax.
Enjoy your new lifestyle.
Appreciate your extra energy.
Notice your improved health.
Learn to accept yourself as you are.**

**The only alternative would be
to do something unreasonable
and push your body to an unnatural size
that could be maintained only
through obsessive behaviors.**

We all know people who talk about food, weight, and dieting all the time. Traditional dieting turns into a full time job that requires all your energy into in order to be successful. Any self-improvement program that is to be effective must help you build a healthy lifestyle that you enjoy and will continue even when life gets stressful. In order to be comfortable with (not compulsive about) your body and your weight, you need to find a relaxed way to think about nutrition that is based on enjoyment, not willpower. You CAN enjoy good nutrition even though you are never going to go on a diet again!

Beware of the "Diet Vortex"

Even though you have decided to avoid dieting, you may still be accidentally sucked in by the "Diet Vortex". You may start out trying to eat more fruits and veggies, and accidentally end up eating more than you really like. In your enthusiasm for healthy eating, you may force yourself to eat things that you don't enjoy, and then you might *feel* like you are on a diet. Some people try the "Exercise in Halves" (where you divide your food in half in order to take a moment to notice if you are satisfied before you eat the other half) and accidentally use this exercise as a tool to stop eating and leave half of the food. Oops, these are dieting thoughts and behaviors.

Decades of dieting experience causes a pattern of thinking that is like a powerful vortex. It can suck you into restrictive eating before you realize it. There is a great difference between dieting that includes restricted eating and this process of healthy eating based on internal signals. It is a subtle difference. It is an important difference.

Carl and the Popcorn

We had been working together for a few weeks. Carl was in his fifties. He had been fat all of his life. After trying every diet and loosing weight time and time again, he found himself fatter than ever. This time he just could not get himself to try another "program". When he read about this healthy eating based on *enjoyment* rather than on willpower, he had to try it out. He was thrilled with his first exercise: "Savor Your Food". He tuned in and experienced what he ate. When he was satisfied, he asked himself the question, "Why eat it?" As he answered that question, he began to learn many emotional reasons he ate. He became aware of his emotional needs that used to motivate him to eat. He thought of those needs and chose other ways to meet them. He was using food less. This was good.

******

If Carl were able to achieve these goals, he would not eat more than was comfortable. He would find an amount of food that his body needed to be healthy. That is what is supposed to happen. However, almost everyone, including Carl, temporarily veers away from these simple new goals and slides into more familiar goals of the past.

After a few weeks of working toward healthy eating, Carl reported that he was beginning to crave popcorn every evening. When he ate it, he savored it, but it still tasted good all the way down to the bottom of the bag. He had started eating a bag of popcorn every night. Something was going on. As we talked in our weekly session, Carl started to blame himself. He said, "I am sabotaging this one just like I have sabotaged all the rest." Did you hear it? Did you hear what he said? I did. Carl was talking about this process of healthy eating *as if it were a diet.*

Carl had been sucked into the diet vortex. It happens. After years of dieting, even though he was trying something different, Carl had accidentally started to act like and think as if he were on a diet. He had started to use diet goals and diet motivations. Even though he was savoring his food, he was using "Savor Your Food" as a tool to force himself to eat less. He was eating smaller breakfasts. He was doing "real good" and avoiding snacks. He was eating low fat at lunch and dinner. He was eating only fruit for desert. He had put himself on a diet! And, funny thing, he had the exact same reaction that he would have had IF he were on a diet. He began to get cravings and experience binges.

What is the solution? How can Carl get out of the diet vortex? My answer seemed almost too simple: "Focus on the new goals of this process."

- eat nutritious foods when you are hungry
- experience and enjoy what you eat
- stop eating when you are satisfied
- meet your emotional needs without always using food

It is simple, and effective. I suggested that Carl add foods to his meals that might be more satisfying. Protein digests more slowly than carbohydrates, so perhaps if he ate a little more protein at meals he would reduce cravings. Next, I suggested that Carl notice when he was hungry and **EAT whenever he was hungry**. Fruits and/or veggies would be a great choice for snacks. How much should he eat? I don't know. Carl's body knows. I suggested he eat until he feels comfortably full or satisfied. Instead of trying to trick himself into eating less, Carl should focus on his own feelings of satiety. He should eat healthy foods until he is satisfied. Yep, I told this fat man to eat more healthy food, listen to his internal signals of satiety, experience and enjoy popcorn if he wanted it, and stop eating popcorn whenever he was satisfied.

That is just what Carl did for the next week. He reported that he had only had popcorn on two evenings. He only wanted half of the bag. He could see how the old diet goals of restricting food had actually *caused* him to eat more. He calmed down and focused on the specific, constructive goals that we had set in our session. These goals were enough to keep him busy. He was surprised that thinking about these new goals took up all his attention. He did not have to try to avoid the dieting goals. He just needed to **increase** his focus on his new healthy lifestyle goals. The next week he did not happen to want popcorn at all. He could have had all he wanted.

Chapter Three

Fitness and Motivation

The Time of Your Life

Each day,
      each week,
            each month,
                  each year,
They pass by like snowflakes falling.
Falling peacefully, silently, at times,
Sometimes roaring past with a howling wind.

What difference does a little snow make?
Such a tiny thing, a snowflake.
They float past you as if they don't matter.

They matter. Turn around. Look behind you.
That mountain of snow fell one flake at a time.

Are you playing in the snow?
Do you have sleds, and snowshoes, and boots and gloves?
Get what you need and go out and play!

This is the time of your life.
It is up to you. It matters … YOU matter.

A Dangerous Myth

Do you believe you are totally responsible for your body size? If you think you only need to try hard enough and you will reach your "goal weight", then you are the victim of a dangerous myth.

Body size is determined by many factors. You *do* have control of *some* of these factors (like building a comfortable healthy lifestyle that is not some rigid "program".) *You do not have control of many other factors that determine body size.* Therefore, you are not responsible for your body size. You are responsible for the lifestyle you build for yourself!

People with healthy lifestyles come in all sizes!

**If weight loss is your primary goal,
every act becomes an exercise in self-criticism.**

**When healthy living is your primary goal,
every act becomes an exercise in self-nurturing.**

The myth that we have the power to control our body size has caused much pain and suffering. Don't be a victim of the myth. Don't teach this myth to others. There *is* something you can do to stop being a victim of this myth.

**Build a comfortable healthy lifestyle
because you deserve to take care of yourself,
NOT to lose weight.**

You are responsible for your behavior. You are **not** responsible for your body size. You can find peace of mind and wellness, whatever size is natural for you. You can encourage others to do the same.

Please Don't Exercise to Lose Weight

There she was. Five feet tall, weighing ninety-eight pounds soaking wet. And she was soaking wet. She was the aerobic instructor at my local spa. Most of the participants in her class were either young or thin or both. I began to understand why as I listened to her talk: "This exercise will flatten your tummy. This one will smooth out those unsightly bulges in your thighs. And if you keep up with this exercise, it will lift your sagging breasts." Anyone who is not thin or not young knows all this "body shaping" is a lot of bunk!

Please don't exercise to lose weight! If you exercise to lose weight (and if you are normal and your body's own set point prevents you from maintaining that weight loss), then you would be likely to stop exercising because it did not work. It *does* matter *why* you exercise. Your motivation is the strongest factor in choosing to continue or to stop exercising. Nobody wants to keep working toward an unattainable goal.

Please don't exercise to lose weight.
If you exercise to shrink or erase some part of yourself,
then every session would become a mental exercise
in self-criticism and body loathing.

Exercise to take care of yourself!
When you exercise in order to take care of
the wonderful body that nature has given you,
then every session becomes a
mental exercise in self-nurturing.

Move your body because your body deserves
to be taken care of, whatever your size or shape.

The truth is that being in shape has ***nothing*** to do with the shape of your body. Fitness is the result of your actions, not your body size. What actions do you need to take to be fit? There are three components to fitness. Anyone, any size, any level of mobility, can accomplish all three (with some creativity and determination.)

1.) Move rhythmically until you breathe heavily (no mystery, *any* activity that burns oxygen *is* aerobic activity.)
2.) Tone your muscles by pushing or pulling weight in a controlled manner (lucky for us our body weight is available for this task!)
3.) Relax and stretch out those warm muscles, ligaments, and tendons.

When you include these actions into your lifestyle on a regular basis, you have built a fit lifestyle for yourself. Your actions count. So do your thoughts. Don't criticize your body as you exercise, appreciate it.

Appreciate the strong bones that hold you up. Be astounded by the miracle of engineering in your joints. Notice the cooling system that nature has designed for you as you sweat. Marvel at your heart and lungs as they feed oxygen to your muscles. Feel the wonderful muscles that move your bones and support your softness.

Now, what about your softness? It is as much a part of you as any other physical characteristic. Your softness should be considered an asset in your fitness program. Do you have large upper arms? Fine! Those large soft upper arms provide exactly the resistance you need to work your shoulders, upper back and chest. Do you have a round belly? Then use it. Your round belly can work like expensive exercise equipment to provide resistance for working your legs, back, and hip flexors. Your body is not the problem. Your body is the solution to getting more fit, more comfortable, and more mobile!

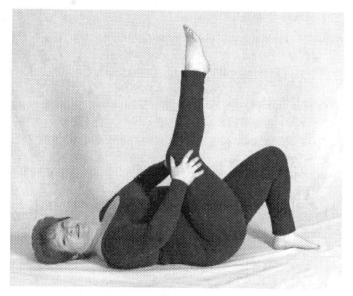

Exercise to improve the function of your body independent of your weight

Keep moving because your muscles get strong when you move. Stretch out because stretching helps you feel better and be more comfortable. Work your abdominal wall because a strong abdominal wall helps prevent low back pain. Develop the muscles that support your good posture because you deserve reduced neck strain and more room in your chest cavity to breathe.

Don't do anything to lose weight. Do everything to keep moving and enjoy your life! Exercise because you deserve to appreciate and take care of yourself.

The Audition

I am angry. I am angry at an idea that causes pain. An idea persists only if people and organizations perpetuate it. So, right now, I am angry at the fitness industry for promoting the "ideal" body as evidence of health and good character. I remember an experience in the early 1980's that left me face to face with this harmful myth.

We all piled into the station wagon wearing our brightly colored leotards. We were on our way to audition for the position of aerobics instructors for Jazzercise™. As we rode down the highway, I thought of the first time I was preparing to go on stage in a leotard. That was the first time I had dieted. That was also the beginning of an all consuming eating disorder that lasted thirteen years. It took years of hard work, but I recovered from bulimia. Here I was again in my leotard, at my natural weight, 127 lbs. I was free from dieting, bingeing, laxatives, diuretics, and vomiting. I felt good.

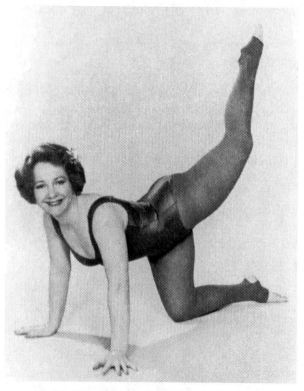

My Jazzercise Audition Photo in 1979

My hard-earned feeling of fitness and confidence was shaken as I trained for this audition. I began to feel uncomfortable about the focus on body size in the training environment. As the day of the audition unfolded, I could not believe what happened. Let me introduce you to the women on this journey with me. One of the trainees was recovering from anorexia nervosa. After a life-threatening low weight of seventy pounds, Cleo was back up to ninety-five pounds. She confided that she still felt fat. However, she was determined to win over this killer disease. Bridget, who was also a trainee, was a very shy person. She had developed her teaching style in harmony with her shyness, not in spite of it.

So, there were three of us, Cleo, Bridget, and me. After a tension-filled ride we arrived and the audition began. The evaluator watched and took notes as we performed. Then one by one, she met privately with each of us. I went first. As I returned to the group after the meeting, I applied my smile. Each trainee left and returned smiling and silent. It was not until the ride home that Bridget (the shy one) announced excitedly that she was accepted as a trainee instructor.

Bridget was told she would have to work hard these next three months if she wanted to be ready to become a full instructor. The evaluator did give her some advice: "Go to as many classes as you can, and stand near Kelly. Watch her, and try to move like her." Cleo (95 pounds) was not accepted. She had asked what she could do to improve. She was told: "Look at Kelly. She is not as tall as you are, but her movements are bigger. She has energy with control. Watch her, then work with yourself in a mirror." Cleo and Bridget talked excitedly as they began to schedule classes. "Which classes can we attend, so that we can prepare together to be full instructors?" they asked me. None. I would not be preparing, because I was not accepted.

The evaluator was direct when we met. After my performance, before I could even sit down she said, "There is only one reason that I am not accepting you." Yes? Yes? "You are too fat." But...but, how were my execution, my enthusiasm, and my teaching style? Her answer, "Great! On those points I would accept you on the spot."

Questions raced through my mind. Yes, there was some important information that I wanted from her. Other than my body size, what did she think I needed to change? She replied, "You don't need to change a thing about your performance or your teaching. What you should do is this. Stand naked in front of a mirror. I know that this is hard." (She did not know how hard I had struggled and that I like the way I look in the mirror.) "Now," she continued, "look at those bumps of fat that shouldn't be there. Then as you sit down to eat, remember those bumps, and eat accordingly."

I know only moments passed before I spoke. It seemed longer. On this day I was not going to be the victim of this evaluator's size prejudice. I had no interest in working for a company that supports these views. I thought of the other women who are about to talk to this evaluator. I had to say something. I needed to tell her about some of the harm she could do if she gives this well-meaning and dangerous advice to others.

I took a deep breath to calm myself. I told her that I could not believe life has given me another chance at the same scene. But here I was, listening to *exactly* the same advice that was the foundation of my eating disorder. She listened as I continued. I told her that I had already been the victim of the "really look at yourself critically" method of weight loss. When I looked in the mirror and cultivated a disgust for my "problem areas", I began to have a distorted mental image of myself. I could not see my whole self in the mirror. I only saw parts of myself, a hip, a belly, a thigh. I was growing farther and farther away from the natural feeling of eating from hunger. I was developing a response to my distorted view in my mirror. Then I would eat, or vomit, accordingly.

So please, I told her, do not give this pathological advice to anyone else. The most common result of this "critical look in the mirror" is to distort a person's body image. A more serious result is that you would be contributing to the epidemic of anorexia and bulimia in our society today.

This dance exercise company, and most other fitness companies, promote the myth that anyone can have a lean body if they exercise enough. Hiring only lean instructors reinforces this idea that only lean bodies are fit and that only thin bodies are healthy. An army of lean instructors has a message to the average person. "If you do not look like us, then you have not tried hard enough."

What if, no matter how hard a person tries, it will never be enough to battle his/her own body's natural size? What are the consequences of trying? There is considerable evidence that this weight loss and weight gain cycle **is** the cause of many health problems usually associated with fatness.

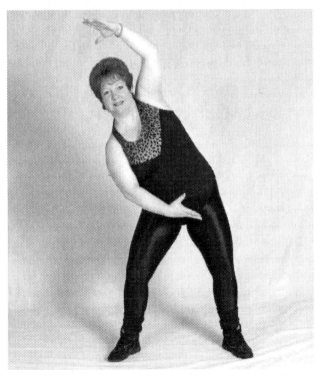

My fitness photo in 2000

I believe that people are supposed to come in all shapes and sizes. Everyone, of any size, has the right and responsibility to work toward fitness. Fitness is the result of a healthy lifestyle. When a person works out regularly and effectively, they may still remain fat.

Fitness has <u>nothing</u> to do with fatness. That is why I opened my own exercise studio shortly after this audition. My studio financed my advanced fitness certification and my graduate degree in education.

You can help to end size discrimination by asking for full-figured instructors at your health clubs and gyms. You can demand classes for people of all sizes that focus on improving fitness and healthy eating, rather than promoting thinness. You have the power to help by seeking out and supporting businesses that provide service, without incrimination, to people of all sizes.

When it Comes to Fitness, What Do I Want to Give Myself?

This is not a selfish question. This question helps you take better care of yourself. When you feel better and have more energy, you can be more effective in your life, your family, and your community. Ask: "What do I want to give myself today that will help me feel my best?" With so much to do, it is tough to find time to take care of yourself. Sometimes it even seems selfish to spend any time on yourself when so many others need your attention. You will be able to do more for your friends and family when you meet your basic needs first. The truth is, if you take care of yourself, you will get more done in the long run.

One of your body's basic needs is for regular movement. Whatever you do in your busy life, you and your body will be doing it together. It is so tempting to say, "I'll wait until after things calm down to get back to my fitness". Don't wait. It costs too much. Life is complicated. You may end up waiting for months before things calm down. You deserve to feel your best. You should be able to enjoy higher energy. You need the stress relief that comes from regular movement and exercise!

Think about how you feel as you face a busy day or hectic time in your life. What do you want to give yourself today? You might want to feel better or have more energy so that you can do the jobs ahead of you. If you need more energy, do something active. Get your circulation going. You will feel better. The weather may prevent you from going outside. Do something inside. Put on your favorite music and dance. (You can boogie in a chair if you need to.) If you have in-laws visiting and you don't want to dance around your house, dance around your bedroom using headphones.

If you usually use weights for muscle toning, you may not have any available when you travel. Pick up a book, a bottle of shampoo, a small bag, and try some muscle toning moves with these substitute weights. If you can't get to the gym, pretend your bed is your exercise mat. Almost anything you can do on an exercise mat, you can do on your bed. Many of my clients prefer this soft flat surface to the floor anyway.

When you get to the mall, don't shop right away. Before you load your arms with packages, you can enjoy some mall walking. (I have several clients who use a wheel chair and who enjoy *mall wheeling*.) Start out with five minutes of slower walking in good posture for a warm-up. Next, walk fast enough to breathe a little heavier and you are doing an aerobic workout. It does not matter whether your aerobic walking lasts one minute or one hour. It matters that you listen to your body and end up feeling invigorated, not tired. Finish up with another five minutes of mellow walking for a cool-down. Then, you are ready to start your shopping clear-headed and energized.

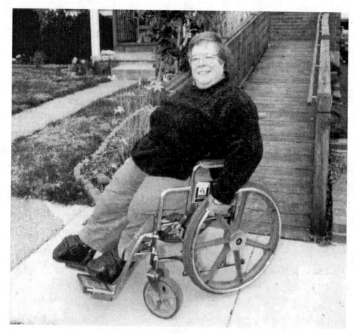

People with any ability or disability can still work out and improve fitness.

Movement brightens your mood. Your cheeks will be pink and you will be warmer. Your joints will be less stiff. Your back will be stronger and less likely to ache. Don't put off movement until after your other tasks are done. Move *first* and you will have more energy to do the rest of the tasks in your day.

Three Clients

"What good will exercise do for me? I will never be skinny anyway." Oh, no, another casualty of "The Lie"! All the advertising shows athletic thin people in the health clubs. The lean and perky fitness instructors look nothing like the average person. The fitness industry tells us that the main reason to exercise is to lose weight. The Lie is that you have to be thin to be fit and healthy.

The truth is that when people have a healthy eating style and exercise regularly, some will be small, some will be medium, and some will also be large.

But, since the truth does not sell health club memberships to a fat-phobic society, they keep telling us the lie.

Wait a minute. If weight loss is not the reason to exercise, what is? The reason to exercise is to feel better and be healthier! To demonstrate this point, I would like to tell you the true stories of three clients. Out of respect for their privacy, I will use fictitious names.

Betty

Betty came into my office at the mental health center downtown. She was an intelligent professional woman who was suffering from a mild depression. She had delayed seeking help because she was afraid of being put on anti-depressant medication. We discussed other alternatives. I asked her if she would be interested in trying a naturally occurring substance provided by her own body, endorphins.

Betty decided to start an anti-depressant exercise program. She added a daily walk to her life. This was not easy. She had to do a lot of problem-solving to fit a walk into every day. Each time she walked briskly for at least twenty minutes, her body would release endorphins. Since endorphins are the body's own natural mood elevators, she felt better. As her depression lifted she was able to make other improvements in her life. But it all started by adding enjoyable movement into each day!

Kathleen

Kathleen did not come to see me. Kathleen did not go anywhere. She was a beautiful super-sized woman who found walking difficult. Life was difficult. Mostly, she stayed in bed watching TV and reading. Kathleen's friend called to ask about a custom-made exercise video for her. I went right into my bedroom, climbed into bed, and started designing a fitness program to be done *in bed*.

Sitting up against the headboard with a cushion at my back, I demonstrated and videotaped exercises for the neck, shoulders, arms, back, abdominal wall, quadriceps, calf muscles, and feet. Then I showed a full body stretch out ... *in bed*.

Yes, Kathleen could do this work. Her TV was right there. Her own personal trainer was available anytime she wanted. Soon I had to design a workout to be done in a chair. Kathleen called her workout "Sitting Aerobics". The next workout using a walker was her favorite. I am planning a freestanding workout at the time of this writing.

I can hear the smile in Kathleen's voice as we have our weekly counseling sessions. She has changed her outlook. She now feels empowered to affect her life!

Doris

That brings me to the last client I wanted to mention in this section. As I was walking down the driveway to my studio, I saw a woman walking ahead of me. I have a long driveway, so I could not see her very well. She had on her short winter jacket with the hood pulled up. The bounce in her step and the youthful curves to her round figure gave me the impression she was in her twenties or thirties. Who could this hooded woman be?

Just then Doris turned around. Doris? Oh, yes. She was scheduled for a personal training session in a half-hour. Doris had been coming to my classes for five years. She had been exercising all of her life. Doris was seventy-six years old! As her bright eyes peered out of her wrinkled face, she told me, "As long as I keep moving, I keep young!"

******

How can exercise make such a difference in the quality of life? Let me tell you some facts about regular exercise. Think about your joints. You know that most of the joints of the body have cartilage. Did you know that your cartilage does *not* have any blood circulating in it? Your cartilage relies on a substance called synovial fluid to provide nutrients and wash away waste products. The only thing that causes your synovial fluid to circulate in your joints is *movement*! That is why we feel stiff when we sit around too much. That is why we have healthier joints when we move.

Now, think about your heart. Yeah, yeah, we all know exercise is good for your heart. But, why? Because your heart beats more slowly when you are more fit. What is so good about a slower heart rate? Blood only circulates through the heart muscle *between heartbeats*. When your heart rate is slower, you have more time between beats. Your heart has more nutrients available and has more waste products washed away. When you are fit, you have improved your own body's ability to strive for optimal heart health.

Finally, think about your life. So often life is filled with things over which we have no control. Sometimes it feels like we are being run over by a truck. Taking action to improve our lives helps us to feel empowered. Feeling like we can have an effect prevents us from being victims. Moving and using our own bodies is one small action we *can* do.

When you add enjoyable safe activity to your daily life, you may be small, medium, or large. You definitely will be healthier and feel better. Many scientific studies have proved that fitness helps people to stay younger, heal faster, and be more able to meet life's challenges.

If you like yourself the way you are, you deserve the benefits of fitness. If you do not like yourself the way you are, you might want to get to know and love yourself through movement.

"I'm weight training!" and "I'm doing aerobics!"

You talk to yourself all the time. Everybody does. Listen to the way you talk to yourself as you go through your daily life. When you get up out of a chair and find yourself straining, you might find that you criticize yourself like this: "Geez, how did I get so big. I can hardly lift myself up. What a slug I have become. Etc." If you hear thoughts like this in your head, welcome to the human race. Self-criticism is normal. It is just not helpful. Thoughts like this will drain away your self-esteem and your motivation to take care of yourself. These thoughts hurt.

The next time you find yourself struggling to get out of a chair, I want you to remember something. When you lift your body weight, and it is difficult, you are exercising your muscles very strenuously. You are weight training. Some people buy special equipment in order to work their muscles. You have your weight training equipment available all the time. Yes, this is a challenge. It is also an opportunity. Next time you push hard to lift your body weight, don't criticize yourself, APPRECIATE YOURSELF. Say to yourself: "I am doing weight training!" When you appreciate your efforts and take pride in the work you do then your self-esteem benefits. You boost your motivation to take care of yourself. These appreciative thoughts help.

Now, think about walking up a flight of stairs, up a hill, or even through the mall. Do you get out of breath? Do you get out of breath walking around the mall? It is so natural to criticize yourself at times like this. Frustration wells up when you want to get from here to there and your breathing will not let you. At times like this, it can feel like you are trapped by your body, like your body will not let you live your life. It is easy to feel bad about your body, your low stamina, your very self. Can't you just feel your energy and hope draining away?

There is another way of looking at the situation. First, I need to give you a definition. "Aerobic Exercise: Any exercise or rhythmic movement that causes the participant to breathe rapidly." Think for a moment about this definition. It does not say that you must be wearing spandex or standing in a health club fitness class in order to do aerobics. It says that anytime you breathe rapidly you are doing aerobics. Yes, whenever you find yourself breathing heavily on the staircase, on a hill, or in the mall, you are doing aerobics. This is a good thing. There is no reason to criticize yourself just because you do your aerobics more often than other people do. You can choose to appreciate yourself for using your muscles so well that you are participating in your aerobic training. And, the more often you let your body experience your aerobic training, the more fit you will become. Gradually, your body will be able to move farther and faster. Yeah, you may breathe heavily when you move around. Good for you! Change the way you think about your body. Tell yourself: "I'm doing aerobics!" Appreciate your efforts. You will feel better. Feeling better keeps you moving.

Three Reasons It Is Tough to Exercise

Anyone of any fitness level at any size can increase his/her fitness and wellness!

How can I say such a thing? I say this because I know it is true. My life has taught me. In 1991 I was in the final negotiations for the opening of my fitness studio called "Work It Out, Inc." On my way to a meeting, I was in a car accident where I suffered a head injury. The medication they gave me to control the resulting epileptic seizures made me sleep twenty to twenty-two hours a day! (I have come to think of this as my larval phase.) I was only awake a few hours each day and I was coping with a major medical problem. I really got a chance to experience the reasons that get in the way of starting or continuing a fitness program.

Reason #1: "I have no time."

In the few hours I was awake, I did my workout **first**. After that, I talked and laughed with my kids while we did household tasks and ate dinner together. Then I took my medication and slept. My training as a psychotherapist and personal fitness trainer told me I really needed to take care of myself if I was going to recover. I was at risk for depression, muscle atrophy, and spinal problems. The only way I could be sure to fit my workout into my day was to do it first thing. (When I think about my clients, the ones who workout early in the day are twice as likely to maintain their fitness program than those who plan to workout at the end of a long stressful day.) Later on when I was feeling well enough, I found that making the commitment to attend a class, preferably with a friend, also helped me to fit the workout into my day. Because my friend was expecting me, I was more likely show up. It was like an appointment. I worked my schedule around my workout class.

Fitness Recommendations
- **Workout early in the day,** before life's complications and exhaustion make it difficult.
- **Workout with a friend if possible**. Even if you workout at home with a video, make room for two in front of your TV. You may be tempted to cancel a workout for yourself, but you will be less likely to cancel on a friend.
- **Join a fitness class, especially if you need to put your workout late in the day**. Your workout becomes an

appointment just as important as any other commitment. Plan your schedule around your fitness, don't just hope to fit it in.

Reason #2: "It has been so long since I exercised. I'm so out of shape, I would not know where to begin."
After my accident, I lost my muscle tone and stamina. I decided to start a walking program right in my neighborhood. When I walked just to the top of my inclined driveway, I was exhausted! I had to go back to some basic principles of fitness in order to progress from completely sedentary to fit.

Fitness Recommendations
- **Select a workout environment that promotes self-awareness and self-regulation of your workout.** Find an environment where you are taught to pay attention to how your body responds to the exercises. You need information on how to modify the moves for your fitness level. You need to be appreciated for pacing yourself. When you select a place to workout, make sure you get encouragement to do your best and information on how to tune in and pace yourself.
- **Always include a warm-up in your routine.** During your warm-up work at whatever level of intensity is mild for you. Tune into how you feel when you move and start out moving at a pace that is comfortable to you. Do not let anyone or anything intimidate you into pushing harder than you should, especially in your warm-up. All those capillaries in your extremities need time to dilate so they can carry oxygen to the muscles during your aerobics. If you skimp on your warm-up you will feel exhausted at the beginning of your workout because of oxygen deprivation to your muscles. Most people who are just getting into shape get more sore muscles than necessary because the warm-up they do is too intense for their present condition!

Reason #3: "I have no energy. My work, the house, my family, and other obligations take all my energy."

When I was on the anti-seizure medications, I had no energy at all. This experience gave me great empathy for my counseling and fitness clients who felt overwhelmed and tired. I was glad for the empathy and understanding, but I still needed more energy to live my life and get well. That is when my logical mind took over. If I have low energy, will I get more energy by being lethargic? I don't think so. If I'm feeling overwhelmed, will I feel better by just sitting around worrying? No. I decided to begin a walking program even though I had little energy. That was one small thing I could do each day that would increase my energy and help me feel in control of something. It worked. I walked for only a few minutes at first. I was persistent. In a few months I was walking a mile. That was enough to release endorphins and other neurotransmitters that brightened my mood. My physical energy increased. I still was only awake a few hours, but I was more hopeful and energetic when I was awake.

Fitness Recommendation:

Exercising regularly, at the proper intensity for your fitness level, gives you more energy for your work, your house, your family, and your other obligations!

I used these very same fitness recommendations in my own life when I was rehabilitating. Getting fit was like a lifeline. My workout was one of the few things I could control. I would not be the victim of my accident. I was the person in charge of my rehabilitation. I started thinking of a way to get back to work. I could work with my psychotherapy clients by phone and I could work with my fitness clients using video! If I had a seizure, I could hang up the phone or turn off the camera and come back later.

I believe that anyone of any fitness level **at any size** can become more fit. I have seen it happen in my life and in my clients' lives. Over the last eighteen years I have seen clients overcome many obstacles to fitness and happiness. My clients and my own rehabilitation have given me hope. Hope is contagious!

A Menu for Movement

When I sit down to make my selection from a restaurant menu, I feel so pampered. I can choose anything I want. I don't have to think of what's available. The list is right in front of me. All I have to do is tune in to what I feel like eating, find it on the menu, and order it. Wouldn't it be nice if more of life were that simple?

Wouldn't it be nice if adding movement and fitness were as easy as ordering from a menu? It can be. You can design your own movement menu. Even if you are sedentary, you have more items on your menu than you think.

One of the most important items on the menu is the Stretch and Relax Workout. This is any gentle stretching routine that feels good. You can stretch out in bed, in a chair, and standing. You can use the stretches you will find at the end of any workout video that you like. You may have a favorite set of yoga stretches. You might just tune into your body and move gently as you feel muscles stretch out. Start at the top and work down, focusing on each area. The goal of this workout is to relax both body and mind.

When you are tired, stretching can revitalize (and does not require energy to do.) If your legs and feet hurt, stretching will encourage circulation and make them feel better. If you have problems with your back, your doctor has probably already given you stretches to do to relieve back strain. Do them. Once you have some stretches that you enjoy on your menu, you have a selection available when you want a break from more strenuous exercise. There is almost no reason not to use your Stretch and Relax workout. You can fulfill your commitment to daily movement *and* rest at the same time.

If you can't walk, get a few videos that show you how to exercise in a chair and on your bed. Start to work out the details necessary for you to get to a pool once a week or so. Talk to a professional who can help with fitness even though you have mobility problems. Remember, the more you move, the more you will be able to move. Unfortunately, the reverse is also true. The less you move, the less you will be able to move. I have never had a client who could not find a way to add more movement to his/her life. You can too.

If you can walk at all, you have a very powerful fitness tool available to you. Even if you have been completely sedentary for years, walking can get you moving again. The key is to start very, very easily and increase slowly. You want to give your body time to get stronger. If you weigh a lot, your weight provides a wonderful fitness tool. You are doing aerobic weight training every time you walk. Tune in to how you feel. Most people expect too much from their bodies at the start. By *gradually* increasing your abilities, you will make the fastest progress in the long run.

Now, think about your basement, attic, and closets. Do you have any fitness equipment that you purchased in the past and don't use? If you do, welcome to the human race! Some of that equipment may be useful to you now. If it is comfortable, enjoyable and accessible you may want to incorporate it into your movement menu. You may want to experiment with the different items to see if you can use them at this time in your life. Perhaps all you need to do to enjoy your reclining bicycle is to put it in front of the TV instead of in the basement. If you like cycling, but get bored on a stationary bike indoors, try riding outside and enjoy the scenery. Try some problem-solving. Most of all listen to your body. If a piece of equipment is uncomfortable, miserable to do, or inaccessible, you may want to sell it or give it away. If you try something and it does not work for you, you did not fail. It just was not right for you.

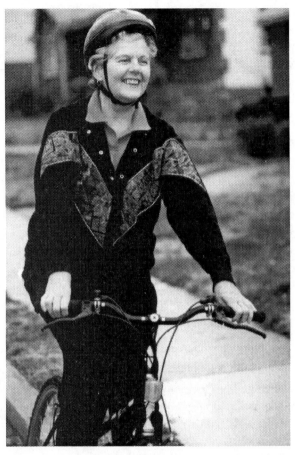

Finding enjoyable fitness puts a smile on your face at any age

What about the activities in your daily life? I know when I mow my lawn I get a steady hour-long aerobic workout. What about you? Vacuuming, raking, and sweeping can be a great workout for the butt, thighs, back, and upper body. Just remember to change sides regularly, and to step forward putting weight on the forward leg (without bending your back forward, which could cause back stress.) This is just like doing eight lunges right and eight lunges left. Notice anytime you find yourself breathing heavily during your daily activities. That means you have found an **aerobic** activity. You can add that to your fitness menu. Do you like line dancing, cycling, hiking, swimming, body surfing, etc.? If it causes you to breathe heavily, it can improve your fitness.

> **Yes, anything (including sex) that causes heavy breathing can improve your fitness. This fitness menu is getting better all the time!**

Many people find that having support and structure when they workout is helpful. If this is true for you there are several ways you can accomplish this. If you are lucky enough to have a size-accepting fitness facility near you, participate in a class once or twice a week. If you cannot find a fitness class at a facility that is respectful of your large body, you can still set up a class for yourself. All you have to do is get one or two friends who would like to join you. You can schedule a regular workout time and use size-friendly workout videos for instruction. Make sure to choose videos that focus getting fit, not on weight loss. (You don't want to criticize your body while you are trying to take care of yourself.) When you all chip in for the cost of the videos, you will be able to afford several different workouts. This will be less expensive than classes elsewhere, and you will have companionship and accountability.

Whether you add movement to your life with friends or on your own, your body will appreciate the effort. Your body functions better and heals faster when you move. Only you can decide what items should be on your fitness menu. It will take some problem-solving and experimentation to find the right combination for you.

Now, how you use your movement menu is very important. When it is time to work out, you can choose anything you want. You don't have to think of what's available; the list is right in front of you. Tune in to how you feel. What do you need? Do you want to be energized, relaxed, or spent? Do you want to feel your power, your flexibility, or your endurance? Just find the movement on the menu that will meet your needs, and enjoy it. You deserve it!

O.K.? So HOW do I Get Moving?

We all know that regular exercise is an important part of good health. You will feel better and improve the functioning of your body in many ways through regular exercise. Yeah, yeah, we all know that, but it still does not make it any easier to do it! Well, here are some tips for you that *will* make it easier for you to get moving.

1.) Don't make a commitment to daily exercise ...Make a commitment to something easier! You do <u>not</u> have to find the willpower to exercise daily. Yes, that is what I said. You do not have to talk yourself into doing your workout each day. **You only have to talk yourself into getting dressed and doing your warm-up.** It only takes about ten minutes to dress and warm-up. It is much easier to convince yourself to this one small task, even if you are tired or stressed or lethargic. Once you are warmed up, you will probably <u>want</u> to do the rest of your workout. When your body gets moving, moving feels good. A body in motion tends to stay in motion. A body at rest tends to stay at rest. Make a commitment to dressing and warming up ... after that your workout will just naturally follow!

2.) You can increase your chances of dressing and warming up tomorrow if you take one simple action today. **Get your clothes together <u>today</u> for tomorrow's workout.** If you workout in the morning, put your sneakers and sweats where you will see them and put them on first thing in the morning. If you go to a class, pack your gym bag or swim bag ahead of time. Once you have already prepared for your workout, you are much more likely to follow through and do it!

3.) The solution is in the structure. If you hope to exercise each day, but the days slip by and somehow it just doesn't happen, welcome to the human race. Life is often unpredictable. Something comes up or time flies by and the next thing you know, the day is over and you are hoping to exercise tomorrow. Over the years, I have seen clients overcome these normal human tendencies using two simple techniques:

- **Give yourself a workout first thing in your day.** This ensures that you will exercise before anything can happen to get in the way. You will also have more energy and a brighter mood to face the challenges of the day.

- **Join a class so you have a regular workout scheduled into your day.** This provides the structure that ensures you will take the time for your daily exercise. You don't have to figure out when you will workout. Your day is structured to include the workout for you!

4.) Human beings are social creatures. You are more than twice as likely to succeed if you include a friend in your fitness plans. If you walk in the morning, walk with a friend or join a walking club at a local mall. If you join a class, get a friend to join with you. There will be times when you might cancel if it was just up to you. When you workout with a friend, you are more likely to stick to your plan because you do not want to let your friend down. Exercising with a friend is a wonderful thing to do for you and for your friend.

Whatever your fitness level, whatever your age, whatever your medical condition, your body heals faster and functions better when you get moving. This is a great gift to give yourself. You deserve to feel better about your body and your life!

At Home and Stretched Out

What if you are just starting out, and any exercise seems intimidating? What if you need to stay in the house for some reason? Perhaps the winter weather or the intense summer heat causes problems for you. These issues can be a real challenge to getting fit or staying fit. However, with creativity, patience, and persistence, you can overcome these challenges.

A good place to start is by paying attention to your attitudes about fitness. Fitness has nothing to do with your age or body size. Fitness develops when you take care of the body that nature has given you, whatever your age, whatever quirks may have developed over time.

When you stay at home, you are functioning in a relatively small space. You tend to make relatively small movements. You often miss the full range of motion of your joints and don't stretch your muscles. It can become a downward spiral. The less you move, the less you are able to move. However, the reverse is also true. Once you get moving, even just a little bit, you will be able to move more. The human body is truly a miracle. Let that miracle work for you!

Think about your morning, after you have taken care of basics and before you get dressed. Think about evening, after you have completed your bedtime routine and put on your nightclothes. These are two perfect times to take a few minutes for a gentle stretch. The key is GENTLE stretch. Your muscles are less flexible when you awaken or are tired at the end of the day. But this is exactly when your body needs the extra circulation and relaxation that stretching provides. Stretch gently on the flat comfortable surface of your bed, so that your movements will be both safe and effective.

Start out with a few ankle circles. Just lay back and prop each calf up on a pillow or two so you can slowly move your ankles around. Do eight ankle circles on one leg and then eight on the other. Repeat this cycle as many times as you want. Ahhh! Can you feel all the muscles in your leg moving? Ankle circles increase the flexibility of the muscles, tendons, and ligaments in your foot and ankle. This flexibility makes your arches more comfortable when you walk, minimizes pain from heel spurs, and reduces arthritis pain. The motion of your foot increases circulation in the legs, which helps relieve discomfort from varicose veins. You strengthen the muscles in your leg and ankle that affect balance.

Next, slowly hug ONE knee while the other leg remains bent with the foot on the bed. If you are not flexible and cannot reach your knee, just use the sheet to help you hug your knee in the direction of your torso. This releases the lower back and stretches the back of the leg. But there is a bonus. Do you feel the stretch between your shoulders as your arms reach down? Can you feel the muscles in your arms contracting as you pull gently on your leg? These stretches should feel good, never hurt. Stretch each leg, one at a time. Then set your legs down one at a time and enjoy the tingling from the improved circulation.

Now is a great time to sit up on the edge of the bed. Lift your ribcage up so that you are sitting in good posture while you do some shoulder rolls. Feel the muscles in your upper back and chest as you use them gently. You will feel the stiffness in your shoulders melt away. To release tension in your neck, again sit in good posture and *slowly* look over one shoulder. Hold that stretch and take a deep relaxing breath. Yes, you will probably yawn at this time. Enjoy it! Stretch the other side of your neck by looking over the other shoulder. Relax and breathe again. Can feel how this stretches all the delicate muscles of the neck and upper back?

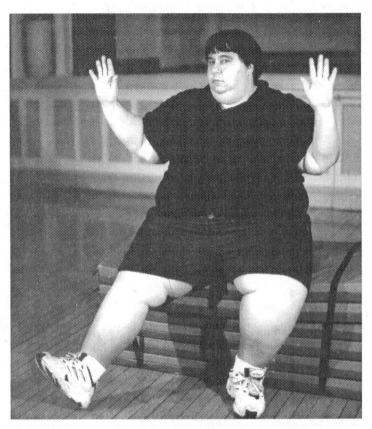

Moving and stretching helps more than your body.
It helps reduce stress too.

Finish off your stretch by reaching your arms out, up, back, around. Reach anywhere that feels good. Reach slowly. Reach gently. Next, place one hand on the mattress beside you and let the other hand reach across in front of you so that you feel a nice SLOW rotational stretch in your spine. Finally, reach both arms up, bend at the elbows, and pat yourself on the back. You have started, or ended, your day with care and respect for the body nature has given you. You are now an active part of the miracle that is unfolding as your body gets more fit!

Stress, Not Always Destructive

Think of the excitement you feel when you are starting a new project that you like and that you know will turn out wonderful. That excitement is a form of stress. It helps you to have the energy necessary to accomplish the tasks at hand. Now, think of the anxiety you feel when you have a job to do that seems difficult or impossible to do. That anxiety is also form of stress.

Alertness and excitement are responses to constructive stress. Anxiety and nervousness are responses to destructive stress. What is the difference? How can we change the way we look at things so that we feel challenged and exhilarated instead of overwhelmed and exhausted? I believe the answer has to do with feeling that you have the ability to affect the situation.

Sometimes it seems like every minute of every day is filled with things that you just have to do immediately. Mornings are hectic as you scramble to get ready for the day. The kids need their boots. The dog needs feeding. The car needs gas. Everybody needs something from you. Whether you work at home or outside the home, your day is filled with tasks that require your attention and your time. After a long day, do you get to rest? No. All the evening's activities and obligations are still ahead of you. Aahh! It is all too much!

You know the feeling; it is like your life is running you instead of you running your life. Somehow, things get away from you and you are reacting to your circumstances. It feels like you have little choice and less control. I believe the feeling of having no control is what causes destructive stress.

Since life is so dynamic and changing, there is no such thing as having complete control of your situation. However, you can feel empowered and hopeful that *you can affect your situation*. When you approach the same situation with a different mind set, you will have a different reaction. As soon as you begin to feel hopeful and able to cope, your reaction to the stress will be exhilaration and energy. By looking at the situation differently you changed destructive stress into constructive stress.

How do I move from overwhelmed to hopeful? There are many ways. I have a friend who meditates when she starts to feel stress. If you would like to use meditation to help you to look at things in a new way, learn more about it. Experiment with it. I have not had much luck; I probably am doing it wrong. I end up thinking about lists of jobs instead of relaxing. So, I have developed a more *active* way to relax. I focus on my body movements and breathing in an exercise I call "Tune In & Chill Out". One of the most important things about this exercise is that it takes less time than going to the bathroom. (No matter what is going on in your life, when you gotta go, you gotta go.) If you have time to go to the bathroom, you have time to:

Tune In and Chill Out
(an active relaxation technique
to rejuvenate and energize)

- Sit on the edge of your chair with your feet flat on the floor for balance and your ribcage lifted in good posture. Relax your neck. Make sure your shoulders are low and relaxed.
- Enjoy slow shoulder rolls, one side, then the other. Breathe in and out deeply as you roll your shoulders. Yawn if you want to. You may start to feel like a cat stretching. Do as many as you want, until your neck is relaxed and warmed-up.
- Next, you will be relaxing tension in your neck area. After you have warmed up your neck and shoulder muscles, sit in good posture again. Inhale as you sit tall. Exhale as you lean your head gently to one side with your ear toward your shoulder. Think about stretching the muscle along the side of your neck. Take three gentle breaths while leaning your head to the side. On each exhale, feel the muscles melt into relaxation. Come back

to good posture and do the same relaxing breathing and stretching on the other side.

Finally, you will alternately stretch between your shoulder blades and release tension in the chest wall.

- **Roll forward:** Start out sitting tall with your hands out at your sides as if you were holding a hula-hoop. Inhale. As you exhale, slide your hands forward along the imaginary hula-hoop until you are rounded forward with your hands together in front and your back rounded. Feel the stretch between your shoulder blades. Take a few gentle breaths, relaxing on each exhale.
- **Stretch up tall:** Inhale as you come up, tracing the hula-hoop back until you are sitting tall with your hands at your sides pressing as far back as possible (that is not very far.) Feel your chest wall stretch as you press your hands back. Breathe gently stretching, relaxing, then come back to good posture. It feels really good to do a few of these "roll forward" and "stretch up tall" in sequence.

When you take a few moments to take care of yourself in some way, you are more likely to be able to cope with the challenges life brings. Just the relaxation and extra oxygen provided by this exercise may change your attitude toward the challenges that you face. Feeling better makes you more hopeful. There are lots of ways you can help yourself feel better even if you have very little time.

- Take a moment to put on hand cream in the middle of a busy day.
- Take two moments and give yourself a hand massage while you are at it.
- Take a five-minute walk around the building or around the block. Breathe. Feel the outside air move past your face. Notice the power of your leg muscles as they

propel you forward. Moving through time and space under your own power can be very therapeutic.

You get the idea. Do something to affect how you feel and you have changed the most important factor in coping with stress, your attitude and your empowerment. Taking care of yourself is worth the time. It gives you more time and energy to take care of everything else in your life.

Why Warm-up?

Once you have decided to add more activity to your life, why is it so important to warm-up before exercise? Some of the benefits of a good warm-up are better demonstrated by a story rather than just explained:

Calista and Me

I was shocked when it happened to Calista and me. We were two young strong healthy aerobic instructors in 1990. We were each teaching many classes every week. We were in the peak of fitness. The classes that we taught were non-impact aerobics. This was VERY unusual for the time. High-impact and step aerobics were all the rage.

We decided to attend some classes taught by other instructors so that we could compare and learn additional moves. Each class we attended was a challenge both physically and emotionally. Often we had to adapt dangerous moves and cope with body loathing comments. However, we could DO the workout. Well, that is, until we went to this one class.

The music blasted, the instructor shouted directions, and the participants were pumped. I felt a bit of pressure to perform. I was the only fat woman in the room and I wanted to prove I was as good as anyone else. (I know that is not the way it "should" be. It was just the way I felt.) I kept pace with every move. I acted like I was fine, like it was fun. In reality, I was in agony. My legs felt like rubber. My muscles burned. I felt exhausted! How could this be? Am I not really fit after all? This isn't that tough a workout. What was wrong?

In the locker room, after everyone else had left, I asked Calista how she felt. She started out saying she was fine and that she enjoyed the class. Then, when I confessed that my legs and arms were killing me for the first half of the aerobic section, she groaned with relief: "My God, me too. My legs felt like they were going to fall off!" We couldn't figure out why this class was so difficult when all the other classes were fine. Were we suddenly out of shape? (I found myself thinking old thoughts like "Am I too fat to do this?") Then it hit us...*We did not warm-up!* The instructor started the class with moves that were fully aerobic, not warm-up moves.

******

Let me tell you what we learned that day. There was good reason for our fatigue and difficulty. I want you to think about all the tiny capillaries that carry the oxygenated blood to your muscles. Your muscles need that oxygen to function. Those capillaries are NOT dilated when your muscles are cold. They cannot carry the needed oxygen to the muscles. The oxygen-starved muscles feel fatigued and burn. You feel like you cannot do your usual workload. You feel weak, experience pain, and have more sore muscles the next day. Missing a warm-up causes problems.

However, when you do warm-up, the capillaries will be fully dilated. The muscles will have more oxygen available. You will be able to function at your best with less soreness the next day. You will feel more successful at your fitness. Feeling successful increases your likelihood of maintaining your fitness for the long haul!

Silly Putty™

Do you remember playing with Silly Putty™ when you were little? When you first took it out of the egg, if you pulled on it, it would snap or tear apart instead of stretching out. But, if you mashed it with your warm little hands for a while until the Silly Putty™ got warm, then it would s-t-r-e-t-c-h out very smoothly.

I would like you to remember Silly Putty™ when you think of stretching your muscles. Cold muscles will be more likely to tear when you stretch them. Once muscle cells tear, the muscle may heal with scar tissue. Scar tissue is less flexible than the original muscle tissue. So stretching cold muscles might actually <u>reduce</u> your flexibility instead of increasing it. Nice warm muscles, on the other hand, will stretch out smoothly and comfortably. You will get maximum flexibility improvement from stretching when your muscles are warm.

This means that you should NOT stretch at the very <u>beginning</u> of a warm-up. You should not hop out of your car at the track, stretch, and then begin walking. Instead, you should hop out of your car and walk at low intensity for a little while until your muscles are warm. Then you can enjoy stretching before you continue your walk. If your fitness instructor insists on putting a stretch at the very beginning of the class, before you have warmed-up, you should arrive at class with your muscles already warm. Your walk from the car will help if you park a few blocks away. Are there any easy gentle aerobic machines that you could use for a warm-up? Take care and warm-up before you stretch. Remember the Silly Putty™ and protect your muscle cells from tearing. Protect yourself from cold stretches.

The goal of your warm-up is to increase your breathing, dilate your blood vessels, and to actually warm the muscle tissue. Sometimes I work with people who have great physical limitations and who cannot exercise enough to warm their muscles. For some people, even low intensity movements are difficult or cause pain. In these unique situations, we have had good experiences using water to warm the body before stretching. Either a warm bath or a warm shower works well (even if a shower chair is used for sitting in the shower.) This will dilate the blood vessels and warm muscle tissue to prepare for stretching. Often, after this warming and stretching, the person will be able to continue and do other exercises that are of great benefit. People with fibromyalgia, arthritis, chronic fatigue, and other chronic pain conditions will find this technique very helpful.

After the muscles are warm, either from gentle low intensity movement, or from a water warm-up, or some combination of the two, now you are ready to stretch. These stretches after your warm-up and before your workout help to prevent injury from pulled muscles. That is good for you. Another good time to stretch is at the end of your workout when you have used your muscles for rhythmic work, aerobic activity, or muscle toning work of some kind. Your warm muscles will love the stretch after your cool-down. Individual muscle fibers will elongate. Circulation will improve. A wonderful benefit from this improved circulation is that your muscles will recover from exercise faster. Remember it is when you *recover* from exercise that your body goes through the physiological changes that increase your fitness. Therefore, you will get fit faster when you give your warm muscles a nice stretch at the end of your workout and cool-down. Good for you!

Warm-Up: More Information

Warm-ups should be rhythmic movements that use similar muscle groups as your activity will use.

Sample warm-ups:
- Five minutes of regular walking is a warm-up for aerobic walking, treadmill, or stair climbing.
- Five minutes of easy swimming is a warm-up for exercise swimming.
- Five minutes of <u>ANY rhythmic movement</u> at lower intensity is a good warm-up for that particular activity at higher intensity.

When you warm-up, you should start out breathing gently and gradually increase your breathing. If you are a small person, you will move more in order to get your breathing and heart rate up. If you are a large person, remember that you are doing weight training every time you move. Respect the work your body is doing. You may need to start out very slowly in order to have an effective warm-up. If you are just starting to get fit, you may need to walk very slowly for your warm-up and walk at a medium pace for your workout. Listen to your own body by noticing your breathing. Listen to your own internal pacing. Do not strive for some specific speed or try to keep up with anyone else.

Interval Walking

How can I get fit *faster*?
How can I make my workouts more interesting and fun?
How can I tune in to my body instead of watching the clock?
How can I shorten my workout time, without sacrificing quality?

The answer is INTERVALS !!!

What is an interval? That is simple. An interval is a workout pattern that includes high intensity and then medium intensity. That's all. Not complicated. Just work harder for a while, and then when you need a break, work medium for a while.

How do I know when to work harder and when to back off? Your body will tell you! There is no magic number of minutes to each interval. You do NOT look at a clock. You just listen to your body.

- When you are working at higher intensity and your body tells you that you need a break because you are out of breath, or feel discomfort in your shins, or it is difficult to maintain your good form as you exercise, then it is time to take a break.
- When you are working at medium intensity and your body tells you that you have recovered, then it is time to kick it up a notch and go back to working at higher intensity.

You can include intervals in any type of workout: swimming, biking, lawn mowing, dancing, walking, etc. Whatever activity you are enjoying, change the pace of your activity based on how you feel. Work harder for a while until you need a rest. Then work medium for a while until you have recovered. Then work harder for a while until you need a rest. (When you think about it, isn't this exactly what we do when we have sex?)

Exercising in intervals is a cycle. The cycle is based on internal motivation. You look inside yourself to notice how you feel. You make every choice based on how you feel. There is no external measure or goal at all. Do exactly what feels good to you. Listen to the expert. The expert on you is YOU.

Here is an example of a fitness walk using intervals:

First: Warm-up by walking slowly until you feel a bit warmer and are breathing a bit faster. This usually takes about five minutes. Do not skimp on your warm-up! A good warm-up makes the entire workout more comfortable and more effective.

Then start your intervals: Each interval has two parts

Part 1: Walk at a medium intensity for a while. Medium intensity means you can pass the "talk test". You can talk `while you walk, but you need to take a big breath between phrases. Notice how you feel. Medium intensity is not a challenge. Medium intensity is comfortable. If you need to go slow to find your own individual medium intensity, that is fine. When you have found your own comfortable pace where you pass the "talk test", remember how it feels. You will use that same pace again.

Part 2: Now you are going to walk as fast as you can for as long as you can. This is the high intensity part. Again, listen to your body. Walk as fast as you can staying in good form and posture. There is no set speed. You have to *listen to how you feel* to decide what is high intensity for you. Stay at high intensity as long as you can. That may be minutes or seconds. That's O.K. When you need a break, go back to medium intensity. Stay at medium intensity until you feel comfortable again.

That is one interval. You can repeat this pattern as many times as you and your body feel are right for you. I have given walking as an example. You can also use interval training with swimming, biking, exercise videos, even housework or yard work.

Remember that you should *never* feel chest pain. If you get chest pain, cool-down and see your doctor. If you get "a stitch in your side", drop down to moderate or low intensity until it subsides.

Finally, cool-down! Walk slowly for at least five full minutes! Your cool-down is VERY important. Your cool-down is necessary for your safety *and* to get full benefit from your workout. That's all there is to interval walking, your internally motivated workout.

Cool-Down: More Information

Your cool-down can be the same activity as your warm-up. If you were walking, walk slowly for your cool-down. (Actually, you can use walking as a cool-down for almost any activity if you prefer.) If you were swimming, then swim at a slow and leisurely pace for your cool-down. On fitness videos, there should always be a cool-down built right into the workout. If you use fitness equipment, you may feel comfortable to cool-down with a very low-key modified version of the activity. However, you may feel more comfortable if you get off of the machine and cool-down by walking around the house or doing the cool-down from a fitness video. At any good fitness club, every workout should be followed by a cool-down.

Now, you may ask, why all this fuss about a cool-down at the end of a workout? Because it is essential to your comfort and your well being. If you workout and then feel stiff and sore, you will be less likely to workout tomorrow. (Even people who cope with chronic pain from fibromyalgia or arthritis or other conditions that result in almost constant pain, will feel LESS pain after a workout when they do a quality cool-down.) There are good reasons that doing your cool-down will make you more comfortable, reduce pain, and increase your well being. It may also help you to get fit faster!

I have something outrageous to tell you. The following statement, however outrageous, is true: You do not get fit from exercising. That is right. Exercise is not what increases your fitness. Exercising taxes your muscles and your ability to use oxygen efficiently. That is good. But, that is not what makes your body more fit. If you do not get fit from exercise, what actually does increase your fitness?

RECOVERY from exercise is what increases your fitness.

Yes, it is when your body **recovers** from exercise that you undergo the physiological changes that are indicative of improved fitness. Your muscle cells are able to use oxygen faster and more efficiently, resulting in increased stamina. When exercising, your muscle cells are challenged by lifting, pulling, or pushing weights (often your body weight.) As your muscles recover from this challenge, your muscles get stronger. Keep in mind that your body actually goes through the physiological changes that result in increased fitness as you RECOVER from exercise. Can you see why your cool-down helps your fitness so much?

The cool-down begins the recovery process. Often, when you workout, lactic acid builds up in your muscles. This can lead to sore muscles the next day or two after your workout. When you cool-down properly, you encourage circulation. This improved circulation can help wash away the build up of lactic acid. A good cool-down can help you to have FEWER sore muscles because you are left with LESS lactic acid in your muscles.

When you workout, your blood vessels dilate in order to send more oxygenated blood to your working muscles. This is especially true of the tiny blood vessels called capillaries. If you workout and then just stop, the blood vessels remain dilated. This can be a problem, especially in the lower extremities. When your blood vessels remain dilated it can cause blood to pool in your feet and legs. At the end of your workout, you need to cool-down so that your blood vessels can return to normal size.

What if you skip your cool-down? Your blood vessels would be dilated. Gravity would pull the blood downward. There would be a lot of blood in your lower extremities. How would that blood get back up to your heart and lungs? It would travel through your veins. There are no muscle fibers in the walls of the veins. Your veins cannot "squeeze" the blood back up to your heart and lungs for fresh oxygen. Your veins rely on the rhythmic contraction of the muscles around the veins to help circulation. The rhythmic motion of the muscles around your veins is what helps send the blood back to your heart and lungs. If you skipped your cool-down, your veins would remain overfull with blood and could become distended. This could exacerbate or contribute to varicose veins. Even if your veins are normal, this pooling of blood is not good for you.

Some reasons to cool-down:
- Begin the recovery process that increases fitness
- Help wash away lactic acid and reduce muscle soreness
- Help tiny blood vessels like capillaries to return to normal size
- Prevent blood pooling in veins of legs and feet
- Increase circulation of blood back to heart and lungs

Ways to Workout

There are many, many ways to get moving. I will comment on a few. I encourage you to get your creativity going and add to the list for yourself. Every body, every size and shape, every ability or disability, **every body can get moving**. Remember that it is not a simple process to include movement in your life. However, you CAN take one step at a time to gradually overcome the obstacles and get moving. Here are some ideas for ways to workout:

1.) If You Can Walk, Then Walk.

We often hear experts say; "Walking requires no special facilities and no special equipment." This is an oversimplification. That's a problem. If you think a task is simple, and it is really complicated, then you are not likely to succeed. You will probably blame yourself. So let's get real about walking as a workout. When you realistically look at the obstacles, you have the best chance of overcoming them.

When you walk: Finding the right time in your day to take your walk is important. I find that my clients who walk first thing in the morning are twice as likely to continue walking as people who plan to walk in the evening are. That does not mean that you must walk in the morning to be successful. It just means that it gives you a better chance. I have found the best thing about a morning walk is that it starts your day off on a positive note. You start your day FEELING yourself move through time and space. You FEEL yourself make physical progress through your world. Also, you do not have the stress of figuring out when you will take care of yourself and exercise. You already did it.

If your schedule requires that you walk in the middle or at the end or your day, you will need to give yourself specific structure to avoid skipping workouts. The reason you need structure if you are going to walk during your day is that "stuff happens". It is too easy to say that you will walk later. Pretty soon later is the end of the day and you have missed your workout. Plan to walk at a specific time.

Many people find that walking during the first half of the lunch hour works well. Some people walk after work or later in the day. I had a client who walked out the door of his workplace and just kept walking. (He did not just walk away from his job. He walked toward his fitness.) He kept walking. Every evening he just kept walking, for a half-hour to an hour, until he found himself back at his workplace parking lot. Then he got in his car and drove home. He said that he arrived home relaxed, decompressed from work, and ready to appreciate his family (and his dinner.) He has been walking for years now. With the money he saves by not joining a gym, he and his wife go on a tropical vacation every winter.

For your well being, I recommend working out on most days. Of course, there are many ways to workout. You may want to check back to the section called "A Menu for Movement" that is earlier in this same chapter. If walking is your primary choice for exercise, you can start out walking twice a week. That is enough to feel a difference in your fitness but not overwhelm your schedule. Once you have started working out a few times a week, you are ready to start asking yourself an important question:

Did I workout yesterday?
If not, then I WILL workout TODAY.

If you did workout yesterday, you can choose whether or not you want to workout today. By asking yourself this question (and working out today if you did not workout yesterday) you will not drop the ball and accidentally miss several day's exercise. Gradually, as you get your life adjusted, you can increase your walking from a few days a week to most days of the week. If you are mixing walking with other exercises, you can gradually increase until you are doing some exercise on most days.

How you feel when you walk: What matters most is HOW you feel when you walk. Where you walk is important to your success. Many people feel comfortable walking anywhere. The park, a neighborhood, downtown, the seashore, for some people it does not matter. If you are one of those people, you are lucky. Enjoy your walk on any level surface available. For others it is not so simple. For many people who have been taunted about their body size when in public, walking around in public places is not a comfortable experience. Even if nobody says a word, some potential walkers might feel uncomfortable (in our weight prejudiced culture) about what people who see them walking might be thinking.

This is not paranoia. This is a reasonable response to an unreasonable prejudice. The only way I know around prejudice is to fight it. First, I will comment on fighting the prejudice that is found in the culture. (Next, I will comment on getting the prejudice out of your own head.) One way to fight negative attitudes toward large people is to do what you want and not let those attitudes stop you. I have seen many clients do just that. They went out and walked, regardless of what others may have been thinking. Soon the prejudiced thoughts of others were irrelevant and did not matter to the walker who was enjoying moving through time and space. Often, the large walker was joined by other people who wanted to walk but might have previously been uncomfortable. I have a high school track at the end of my block. In the spring, I see the track filled with lean running athletes for a while. Then, as soon as a few average and large people start walking around the track, there seems to be a consistent increase in plus-size walkers. You could be the beginning of a trend at your location.

What about the bad feelings in your own head that are triggered when you walk? If you have internalized some of our cultures fat prejudice, you can start to get rid of it. If you notice yourself thinking negative things about your fat body, disagree with those negative thoughts. Disagree in full sentences in full paragraphs. Your mind cannot think two thoughts at the same moment. While you are disagreeing with the prejudice that you learned, you are getting some distance from the hurtful thought. See the section in chapter one called "Flipping the Coin: Finding Positive".

Sometimes, when walking is more difficult than it used to be, there is a tendency to criticize yourself. If you notice yourself thinking body critical thoughts, you can change your mind. You can, with effort, focus your mind on appreciating your present effort. You can appreciate what your body CAN do, instead of criticizing for what you can not do.

How you dress when you walk: Another way to reduce negative feelings about yourself is to take care of and take pride in your body. Let's start with how you dress yourself. If you are plus-size you probably have flesh that jiggles. (At the right time, and in the right place, I hope you learn to appreciate and enjoy your jiggling self. There is nothing wrong with flesh that moves! Actually, it can be quite delightful. Jiggling flesh can be like a wave of life, laughter, moving, and being, that stirs through your whole body.) However, when you walk, jiggling can cause discomfort or chaffing.

Let's talk about your thighs. Both men and women have thighs that rub together when walking. You can tell if this applies to you by looking at your pants. If your pants wear out in the inner thighs, then you need this next bit of advice. When walking, wear shorts or tights that are slippery and supportive. For guys, these are sometimes called biker shorts or biker pants. For women they are called shorts, capris, or leggings. There are many fabrics that are slippery, elastic, and supportive. A familiar fabric is nylon spandex. There are others like Cool Max®, Quick Wick®, and others. The important thing is that the fabric helps support soft flesh, prevent rubbing / chaffing, and is comfortable.

If you are a woman, wear a supportive sports bra. If you cannot find a bra that stops you from bouncing, wear two bras. I'm not kidding. You may feel a little claustrophobic at first, but when you are walking, it feels great to walk without bouncing. (You can take the bras off as soon as you are done.) Whether you are a guy or gal, you can have problems with jiggling chest and belly. For guys try a fitted nylon spandex undershirt for support under your T-shirt or sweats. When you tuck your spandex undershirt into your bike shorts or pants you will get double support for your belly. For women, wearing a leotard can add extra support to both belly and breasts. When you add a leotard to your supportive tights or leggings, you get double support for your belly. Over your support layer of choice, you can wear any T-shirt, sweatshirt, or pants you want. You can choose baggy or fitted. There are no rules except your comfort. You can cover-up or uncover. It is up to you.

With your chest, belly, and legs supported, finally I want to comment on shoes. Even if you are just walking a short distance, it is necessary to have shoes that support your arches, stabilize your feet, and absorb shock. It is time to get new shoes when your heels start to wear on the outside or your foot slides to the outside of the shoe. Wearing quality shoes that are not worn out may prevent an injury. Your feet are the foundation for your whole body when you stand or walk. You need good shoes. Occasionally, I work with a client who is very large and who has stopped wearing shoes because it is too difficult to find shoes that fit. Especially if you are large or very large, you need the support of shoes that fit your feet when you walk. *If you stop wearing shoes, you will probably soon stop walking. Especially if you find it difficult to wear shoes, you need good shoes to keep your mobility.* Even if you never leave the house, you need good shoes.

"House Walking"

This is a workout for those who have mobility problems and those who want a gentle workout right in their own home. I will describe a walking program developed by a creative client and myself in answer to the challenges of limited mobility and back problems. We started out talking by phone because she could not walk to appointments. Now she gets out often and even comes to our fitness class occasionally. When at home, she works out daily to maintain her hard won mobility.

It all started because Sharon had back pain and knee problems. She wanted to get more fit, but she could hardly walk. She purchased and used the "Fitness with Bliss™, Sitting Aerobics" workout video for people who face super challenges to fitness. This sitting workout helped her overall fitness level and reduced some of her back pain, but it did not do enough to strengthen the muscles that help her walk. We needed to add something else to her workout.

Because of her back pain, Sharon avoided carrying any large loads. In one of our phone counseling sessions she was talking about how difficult it was to do the simplest household tasks. She would have to put the laundry away one small pile at a time instead of carrying a basket. She had to carry one object at a time when straightening up a room. As I listened, it sounded like Sharon (the woman who had trouble walking) was walking quite a lot just to do her daily tasks! When I pointed that out to her, she began to feel proud of her accomplishments instead of frustrated by how long it took to get things done. We developed a workout we called "house walking".

The first focus was walking in <u>good posture</u>. This develops the muscles that support good posture in general. Next, it was important to bend and lift with back safety in mind, even when lifting small objects. And finally we had to pay attention to turning around in a small space. For all people, but especially for large people, *it is dangerous to twist or turn on a weight bearing leg.* That is, if you are standing on your right foot and you twist on your right leg, you would be putting potentially dangerous stress on the right knee. In a small space, like in the house, there is a temptation to twist when turning around. Instead of twisting, I encourage picking up the feet and taking tiny marching steps to turn around. This strengthens the walking muscles and minimizes torque or twisting in the knee.

When you put all these together, good posture, healthy lifting, and stepping around when you turn, you can get a good workout while doing daily tasks. The trip from the laundry room to the bedroom may not be as long as a high school track, but it is a lot longer than a treadmill (and a lot cheaper too.) By making many trips back and forth, you will be covering a nice distance. If you apply this same technique to all your household tasks and group tasks together into one nice workout, you are in good shape. You are accomplishing both your household chores and your fitness workout. You will spend a little more time, but you are doing more. This "house walking" workout is especially helpful if you have difficulty walking several blocks at a time. It is also great when the weather prevents you from walking outside.

Walking out in the weather: Do not go walking in the ice or snow. There is too much danger of falling. Do not walk when it is VERY hot. There is too much danger of heat stroke. If you make the right preparations, you can walk outside almost any other time.

Let's consider cold weather walking first. Start walking in the early fall and your body will adjust to walking in the cold as the weather changes. To protect your throat from the cold, your body will efficiently produce a mucus layer. By the time you are done with your warm-up you will have your protective layer in place in your throat and breathing the cold air will feel fine. When it is very cold, you can also wear a scarf over your face. Breathe in through your nose to warm the air, and breath out through your mouth for a quick full exhale. It is up to you to wear coverings on your head, ears, fingers, and face if needed. Dress in layers so that you can take off or put on layers of warmth as you go through your workout. Wear socks (two pairs if needed) that wick away moisture to keep your feet warm. When you start walking in the fall, you will be surprised how well you adapt over the weeks as winter descends. You can enjoy, as the song says, "walkin' in a winter wonderland"

The same body adaptations are true for warm weather walking. If you start working out in spring and continue as it gets warmer, your body will adapt to the warm weather. Every year there are people in my fitness class who are working out for the first time as summer approaches. I hear the veterans of the class tell them it will be fine. I tell them that their bodies will adjust. Still, as the summer progresses, every year I hear the new participants say with shock: "I can't believe it. The heat does not bother me anymore. Not just in exercise class. I mean, the heat does not bother me in my daily life!"

In warm weather choose clothes that will help you keep your cool. If you like to be covered up, there are big mesh T-shirts that let the air flow through and preserve your privacy at the same time. Here is an unusual tip that saved my butt when I was a long distance runner in hot weather: water. Yes, you should drink plenty of water to keep yourself hydrated. And you should not wait to get thirsty, that means you are already dehydrated. So, we all know about drinking water. However my unusual tip is to WEAR water. I'm not kidding. I used to put a wet handkerchief over my head and let it drip onto my shoulders. I held the wet handkerchief in place with a wet sweatband. On really hot days I would wet my shirt before I put it on (I chose printed T-shirts that were not see through when wet) and wear a wet shirt. The other runners were red as beets and panting hot. I could run ten or fifteen miles wearing water and stay comfortable. I am happy to say that I no longer abuse my knees by running. Now, I am the only gardener in my neighborhood who is unaffected by a heat wave. I look silly with my wet head and wet shirt.

But I am calm and cool even when I'm digging a ditch at 99°. If you walk or workout in the heat, try wearing water.

Many pages ago I started commenting on the "simple" exercise of walking. **It isn't really simple at all!** That is important. If you think a task is simple, and it is really complicated, you will probably get stuck somewhere and not finish the task. When you realize the task is complicated and discover the steps involved then you can take those steps one at a time. That is the way to set yourself up for success.

2.) Swimming and Water Exercise

For many people swimming is an ideal no-impact aerobic workout. For others, it is a way to tone muscles and move joints through a more full range of motion than they would be able to on land. If you have mobility problems or if you cope with chronic pain, consider swimming and water exercise as an option.

Using a pool often means that you pack your suit in your bag, change in the dressing room, and enjoy the water. Afterwards there are showers to get the chlorine off your hair and skin. You may want to use a shampoo designed for getting the chlorine out. You may want to use a skin moisturizer to keep your skin in good condition. For many people, that is all they need to do to enjoy water exercise.

However, there are often more obstacles to swimming than you might realize. On several occasions I have worked with clients who had memberships to use a pool, and for some reason, they just did not go. Often the client will even start out the conversation by saying, "This is so stupid. I paid for the membership. It is ridiculous that I just don't go to the pool. There is no reason for me not to go except laziness." Can you hear how this person has called themselves names? Can you see how this kind of thinking actually prevents the person from implementing problem-solving in order to find out what is really going on here? There is always a reason for the things that people do and don't do.

I would like to share a set of solutions with you. As I mention each solution, you will be able to tell what very real problem might prevent a person from going to the pool for fitness. If you do not have any of these problems, then you will not need to try these solutions. If you find that you DO experience these problems and you find that some of these solutions might be useful, remember these ideas and try them out.

Solutions:

- **Buy a suit that fits,** and has the support and coverage you need. Yes, the most common problem that gets in the way of water exercise is having a good bathing suit. With the advent of the Internet, you WILL be able to find the suit you want. You no longer have to rely on local stores. There are businesses on the Internet that specialize in bathing suits of ALL sizes. You are entitled to have a comfortable suit. Go get it for yourself!

- **Get a pair of water shoes.** These shoes are great for protecting your feet from injury or infection. Often the no slip surface around a pool deck is very rough and can actually hurt the bottom of your feet. Another benefit of wearing water shoes is that you won't have to worry about catching athlete's foot. There is another function of water shoes that I only learned about this year. You know those big black stripes on the bottom of the pool? If you ever feel those stripes with your feet, you will find them to be extremely slippery. One of my clients was water walking in the shallow end of the pool. She stepped on a black stripe and her foot slipped out from under her. Because she was in shallow water, she fell with enough force to badly hurt her knee. Whether you choose to wear shoes or not, be careful stepping on those slippery black stripes in the shallow end of the pool.

- **Buy a really BIG towel and bring it with you,** especially in the locker room. You may be comfortable in the locker room. You may be able to walk through the spaces between the benches and the lockers. The locker room at your pool may fit you. But sometimes the towels do not. It can be very uncomfortable to try to dry off with a towel that is too small. (Remember that your body is fine. It is the towel that is too small!) You can solve this problem and feel comfortable if you bring your own fluffy large towel. Wrapping your towel, that you KNOW will fit around yourself, is like giving yourself a hug.

- **Put your suit on at home, if you prefer.** If you have problems with the locker room, don't let that stop you from using the pool. You can put your suit on at home and toss something on over your suit that goes on and comes off easily. For the women, you can use a top and skirt for this purpose (there is less wrestling than with pants.) In the summer, you can get delightful dresses that just toss on and off over your swimsuit. For the men and anyone who prefers pants, you will find that a baggy sweatshirt and sweatpants will work fine in cooler weather. Loose fitting cotton will work fine in warmer weather. Once you are at the pool with your suit on underneath, it will be easy for you to pull off your outer clothes and just enjoy your swim. After your swim, you can towel off with the big fluffy towel you brought and toss on the easy clothes you wore into the pool. Yes, you will still be wearing your damp suit until you get home. Yes, your car ride will be soggy. However, this may cause you to enjoy the next part even more. Just think how delightful you will feel as you peel your suit off in your own room and take your well-exercised body into your own warm comfortable shower. AHHhhhhh!!!!!!!!!

- **Call around and find a pool with steps and railing** instead of a ladder to get in and out of the pool. If you have any problem that would make it difficult for you to use those tiny little ladders, don't apologize for your difficulty. Instead, accept your body and meet your needs. If you need steps and a railing, call around and see if you can find a pool that has them. Some pools even have elevators that are designed for wheel chairs! You may or may not find what you need. But at least you will know that you looked. You never know, if enough people keep asking for steps and railings, your local pool may install them!

You may be able to look within yourself and find other obstacles to swimming or water exercise. If you do, don't tell yourself that those obstacles are "silly" or "foolish" or "ridiculous" (these are words that I often hear people say about themselves.) Instead, accept your reactions as valid. There are real reasons that you feel the way you do. Listen to yourself and understand what gets in your way of water fitness. Then you have a chance of solving the problems so that you can enjoy water fitness.

Types of water fitness:
If you tend to be a solitary person, you may enjoy swimming laps or water walking on your own. These activities leave your mind free to think or to remain blank, whichever feels better for you. If you tend to prefer social settings, you may enjoy water walking with a friend. This is an opportunity to exercise and to talk at the same time. I know several people who have made friends for life in just this way. The key is to tune in to yourself and notice which you prefer, notice what you need. Your preferences and needs may change from day to day or season to season. Pay attention to how you feel. Continue to select a fitness setting that gives you the stimulation or the peace and quiet that you prefer. You increase your chances of continuing your fitness plan by selecting the setting that works for you.

There are many different types of water fitness classes. Find out what is available. You are entitled to try various types of workout and find what you enjoy most. Notice the instructor. Do you feel comfortable with the atmosphere he/she instills in the class? Do you like the music? Pay attention to the speed of movements. Often you can make the movements more comfortable by doing them halftime. Do what feels good to you. If you can find an instructor that shows you how to adapt the move for different needs, that is even better.

Swimming and water exercises can be an important option in your overall fitness choices. Set yourself up for success by paying attention to how you feel and what you need. Important considerations are:

- Do you have the right clothing and gear to feel comfortable?
- Do the pool and the locker room meet your needs? Do they fit you?
- Do you prefer solitary or social workout situations?
- Do you feel comfortable with the instructor, music, and pace?

If you can answer these questions and make effective choices for yourself, you will have the best chance to enjoy and continue your water workouts.

3.) Using Fitness Videos

This can be a way to workout at your own home and on your own schedule. One challenge is to select a fitness video that will not encourage body loathing. Most fitness videos on the market today include negative comments about large bodies and criticism of body shape or texture. I recommend you select a video that focuses on WELLNESS *NOT* WEIGHT LOSS. Avoid body criticism, which can encourage body loathing and decrease your self-esteem. These negative emotions can reduce your motivation toward self-care and self-acceptance. Body criticism can be found in most fitness videos on the market today. Luckily for us, there are more and more self-accepting fitness videos available. If you buy them, then the business owners will be encouraged to make more. If you use these self-accepting fitness videos, then you will be taking good care of yourself in body and spirit.

How can you tell if a fitness video has body criticism in it? Do all the people pictured on the cover look like models? That should be a warning sign. Does the text on the video cover guarantee weight loss, promise body sculpting or shaping, or focus on how this workout will improve your physical appearance? If you see these statements that focus on looks or weight instead of health and wellness, the video will probably include body critical comments that could thwart your self-care and self-acceptance.

As you seek fitness videos that will provide long term motivation, look for plus-size instructors or participants on the cover. If they are depicted as active vibrant people, that is a good sign. Instead of body critical videos, I recommend you choose one of the many size-friendly fitness videos on the market now (there are more on the way every year.) You can find a great list of dozens of videos on www.PlusSizeYellowPages.com   You can also call 1-877-KellyBliss or check out my website www.KellyBliss.com where I have TEN plus-size fitness videos available now with more on the way. Choose a workout that celebrates what your body can DO and how you feel instead of how you look.

Keep looking for a workout that helps you feel better about your body, increases your physical abilities, and helps you function better. These are constructive goals that will encourage self-care in the long run.

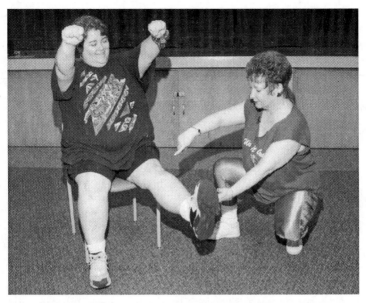

Whether you work out sitting, standing, or reclining, choose the right intensity fitness video for your needs.

Another challenge is how to get started using your videos even when you have them sitting on the shelf. Sometimes people buy a video and have difficulty getting started using it. This is a technique that has worked with countless clients. It may work for you. This is a silly - yet very effective - way to get started. DON'T DO THE EXERCISES. Yes, that is what I said. If you have been resistant to doing the exercise video, then stop pushing yourself. Don't DO the exercises. See if you can PULL yourself toward moving because you WANT to move (instead of pushing with willpower.) I suggest you get a nice drink and sit down and WATCH the video workout. This is a much smaller task. It is much more doable. When you see the workout, you will probably be motivated to participate. Or maybe this time you will watch the entire workout. This may be just the reassurance you need to set aside your fears about the workout. Next time you will know what to expect and it may be easier to get up and move. (Note: if you can tell the workout is not the appropriate intensity, get a different workout so that you can FEEL comfortable.)

4.) At Home Fitness Equipment:

They can be found all over the place. The most expensive clothes racks ever purchased. You have seen them time and time again sitting in the bedroom, spare room, even in the living room, with clothes hanging all over them. (I have even seen them used as plant hangers.) Yes, I'm commenting on home exercise equipment. It is not always that way. It does not have to be that way. I tell my clients who choose to buy home exercise equipment to select items with at least a 90-day return policy. Then, if they are not using the equipment regularly by the time three months have gone by, I suggest they return it.

That is one way to prevent over-expensive overqualified clothes racks from taking over your house. Next, let's consider actually USING home exercise equipment. If you want convenience and privacy for your workout, this may be a good way to meet your needs. Here are some tips that may help you choose the right home exercise equipment for you:

- NEVER BUY FITNESS EQUIPMENT ON IMPULSE! If it is sold now, and it is quality equipment, then it will be sold when you are ready to buy. Wait a few days and take time to prepare for success. If you don't want the equipment after a few days, you did not really want it in the first place.
- BEFORE you go out and spend money on equipment, set up your life and make time for your workout. If you plan to exercise in the morning, solve the scheduling, sleep, and lifestyle issues necessary to succeed at morning workouts. Similarly, for midday or evening workouts, you need to set up your life in order to succeed at fitting

your workout into your day. When you make time in your life for fitness **before** you buy home exercise equipment, you are more likely to use that equipment.

- BEFORE you go out and spend money on equipment, set up your house to make room for your workout. Select your location carefully. Pay attention to how the workout environment feels. Note the view, the light or brightness, and the temperature of the room. Think about other people who live in the house. Will you be able to exercise at your intended time when you consider noise? If you want privacy, can you find a time and place in your home without people watching you. You must have a place to put your home exercise equipment if you are to succeed at using it.

- BEFORE you go out and spend money, try out the equipment that you are considering buying at a health club or at the store. Don't just hop on and see how it feels. Use it. Try using the equipment for **at least five minutes**. How does it feel on your back and your knees? Can you relax while using the equipment? If you feel muscle tension and cannot relax, that tension may cause injury at worst and an unpleasant experience at least. If it is too boring to use for this brief time, you will probably not be able to force yourself to do the exercise for a half-hour at a time.

- BEFORE you purchase equipment, make sure that the equipment you are considering is **rated to hold your weight.** Sometimes you need to pay more for the sturdiness you need. You do not want to workout on wobbly dangerous equipment.

- BEFORE you purchase equipment, think about the type of workout that you have enjoyed in the past. If you liked walking before, consider a treadmill. If you liked working out on weight machines at the health club, try one of the many weight machines using resistance from elastic materials.

- BEFORE you purchase equipment, know yourself. Do you prefer to listen to music, think, read, or watch TV when you exercise? Then choose equipment that will compliment your preference. Will you be able to hear your music over the noise of the machine? Can you put a TV in the same room? If you need quiet to think, is the machine of your choice quiet enough?

After you have thought about and experienced the considerations mentioned above, then you have the best chance of buying the right home exercise equipment for you. After you have purchased your home exercise equipment, use the concepts and tools described previously in this chapter to help you succeed at getting fit.

5.) Fitness Clubs or Health Spas

Select a fitness club or health spa where you "fit in". The most important part of finding a place to workout is your attitude. A constructive attitude to have: If **the health club or spa does not meet your needs, then they are wrong, not you (and not your body.)** Every body takes up space. Small, medium, and large people take up space. Everybody deserves a place to workout where they feel welcome. Members of all sizes should treated with the same respect. Your basic needs should be met.

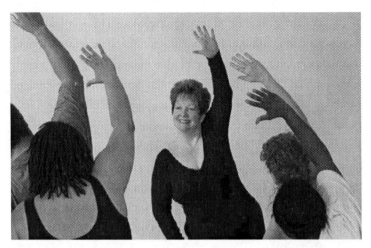

Find a fitness club where you can feel comfortable and the focus is on wellness, not body-critical figure shaping. Here Kelly leads her class in Philadelphia.

As we consider the necessary characteristics of a size-friendly facility, let's start at the entrance. If there is a waiting room, there should be **armless chairs** for large people who don't want to be pinched by chairs with arms. There should be at least one (preferably two) doublewide seats for very large people who do not fit into a single chair. If there are photographs of people working out, there should be fit people of **all sizes** represented.

In the dressing room, there should be room for large and small people to walk between the lockers. The benches or seats should be spaced for the comfort of people of various sizes. (I have had many clients who would love to swim regularly, but the locker rooms are so poorly designed that they cannot walk down the isle or sit on a bench.) The towels should be LARGE. It sounds like a small thing, but it is not. If you are a large person trying to wrap a tiny towel around you, you can't help but feel like you don't fit. That's not true. It is the towel that does not fit. Large towels will make everyone, of every size, feel better. All size-friendly fitness facilities should have large towels.

The staff should be trained to promote wellness, not body criticism and body shaping when they interact with members and prospective members. It would be a good indicator if there were people of various sizes in sales, fitness instructors, and administrative positions.

There should be a variety of low-impact or no-impact aerobics classes offered at several times. The stretching segments should be led by someone who has been trained and/or who has experience in HOW to adapt the stretches to accommodate a round belly. Too often the instructor simply says, "Change the moves if you need to", but does not show (or even know) HOW to adapt the moves.

If there is no health club or spa in your area that meets your needs, don't give up. Call often and ask for what you want. Copy these pages out of this book and mail the information to them. Tell them that it would be <u>profitable</u> for them to LEARN to provide service for the other half of the population. Tell them I will be happy to show them how to make their facility size-friendly. Give them my website **www.KellyBliss.com** and then move on. By asking for what you need and telling your local facilities where they can get the information to provide service to plus-size people, you would have done your part to encourage a size-friendly world. Now you need to build your own size-friendly world.

6.) Workout with Friends:

Whenever possible, whether you are walking, doing aerobics, swimming, using weight machines, using home fitness equipment or videos, try to workout with a friend. If you cannot actually workout with a friend, get a workout phone buddy that you can talk to about your fitness plans and problems. People who workout with a buddy are much more likely to continue to workout.

If you have a workout buddy who works with you in person, then on days when you might not workout on your own, you may workout because your buddy is expecting you. Canceling your workout takes more than just a thought. It takes a phone call to your buddy. That may be just enough to cause you to workout instead of canceling.

If you have a phone buddy, on days when you might not workout on your own, you may workout so that you have something good to talk about when he/she calls. This kind of encouragement and accountability is very helpful for sustaining motivation.

Even though it is statistically true that people who workout with a buddy are more likely to continue in their fitness activities, some people are more simply comfortable working out on their own. If that is you, if you prefer to workout alone, that is fine. You will need to implement problem-solving skills and overcome the obstacles to working out on your own. This is an achievable task. It is a task you CAN do. There are many reasons that fitness is worth your effort.

Sixty Proven Benefits of Exercise

Here is a list of benefits you will receive when you become more active. The organization of the list is from Health Magazine, in their March 2000 issue. The contents of the list could have come from the conversations of people in my exercise classes. Over the years I have heard every one of these comments and more. In our Fitness with Bliss™ classes, we workout in order to improve the function of our bodies and for wellness (not with body critical goals of weight loss). I appreciate all that my class members have taught me about the benefits of fitness.

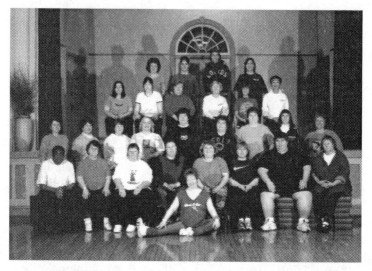

Over the years, class members of "Fitness with Bliss™" have told me of the many benefits they have experienced from getting more fit.

Exercise DECREASES:
1. Bad cholesterol
2. Total cholesterol
3. Other blood fats
4. Risk of dangerous blood clots
5. Heart attack risk
6. Difficulty breathing due to heart disease
7. Illness and absence from work
8. Hospitalizations
9. Risk of colon cancer
10. Risk of developing breast cancer
11. Medical and healthcare expenses
12. Non-insulin dependent diabetics need for medication

Exercise INCREASES:
13. Endorphin production
14. Insulin sensitivity
15. Insulin effectiveness

16. Glucose tolerance
17. Good (HDL) cholesterol
18. The elimination of artery clogging proteins
19. Blood volume
20. Amount of blood being pumped with each beat
21. The chance of surviving a second heart attack
22. Body's ability to use minerals and vitamins more efficiently
23. Lung capacity
24. Oxygen carrying capacity
25. Stamina
26. Bone density
27. Thickness of cartilage in joints

Exercise IMPROVES:
28. Sleep
29. Sense of well being
30. Sense of self worth
31. Joy in life
32. Connectedness with the world
33. Libido
34. Sexual performance and satisfaction
35. Creativity
36. Ability to eat more and gain less
37. Immune system function
38. Circulation
39. Tolerance to heat and cold
40. Posture
41. Efficiency of cardiovascular system
42. Short-term memory
43. Athletic performance

Exercise HELPS:
44. Speed recovery from chemotherapy treatments
45. Anxiety
46. Relieve back pain
47. Overcome jet-lag
48. Alleviate depression

49. Reduce the vulnerability of abnormal heart rhythms
50. Flexibility
51. Lower your resting heart rate
52. Alleviate PMS symptoms
53. Induce relaxation
54. Promote bowel regularity
55. Reduce and prevent menopausal hot flashes
56. Reduce and prevent menopausal sleep disturbances
57. Reduce and prevent menopausal irritability
58. Anger management
59. Relieve and prevent migraine headaches
60. Reduce risk of endometriosis

**Find your own motivation to exercise
from the above list,
or
Find your own motivation inside of yourself.**

(Avoid the body-critical motivation of weight loss.)

Above are 60 positive, self-sustaining reasons to keep exercise in your life. Tune in to your own positive reasons. Write down your own individual reasons. Read your list and own it. Increase your awareness of your constructive motivation so that you will be less likely to get sucked into the body-critical motivation of weight loss. You will see the link between exercise and weight loss everywhere. It is in the media and in the medical recommendations. But you know from your life experience that if you link exercise to weight loss, you will probably stop exercising when you go off your weight loss "program". When you do NOT link your exercise to weight loss, you will be more likely to **KEEP exercise in your life, independent of your weight.**

"Weight loss is not necessary to gain health benefits from exercise" was the headline on November 18, 1999 in NEW YORK (Reuters Health) -- Even if you don't lose weight, you can still gain health benefits from exercising, according to a report presented at the annual meeting of the

North American Association for the Study of Obesity, in Charleston, South Carolina. "Exercise is doing a lot of good whether you lose weight or not," Dr. Steven Blair of the Cooper Institute in Dallas, Texas, told Reuters Health in an interview. At the meeting, Blair presented a review of several scientific studies that show a health benefit in people who exercise but are overweight. Blair said, "Overweight or even obese individuals who are fit have a much lower death rate than normal-weight individuals who are unfit."

Whatever your size, age, ability or disability,
KEEP EXERCISE IN YOUR LIFE,
just because it is good for you,
independent of your weight!

Chapter Four

Putting It All Together

Not as Simple as We Were Told
Or New Goals That Really Work

We hear the same basic simple message from fitness professionals, doctors, counselors, and gym teachers. They learned this basic message from their teachers and mentors. The message is that weight loss is a simple matter of calories in and calories out. Unfortunately, we have all been taught an oversimplified and inaccurate theory.

If body weight were dependent on a conscious manipulation of calories in and calories out, we would all have dramatically fluctuating weights throughout our lives.

**If this simple theory were true, and you ate only
one large apple per day
(that's about 100 calories)
more than you needed, you would gain
ONE HUNDRED POUNDS every ten years.**

This simple theory is not true. The weight maintenance mechanism is much more complicated than calories in and calories burned. Most people do not gain 400 pounds from age twenty to age sixty, even if they eat much more than an extra apple per day. This is not reality for most people. Most people experience *gradual* changes in weight over time.

That is, except for dieters. Some dieters do experience dramatic weight gains in short periods of time. I often work with very large people who weigh between 300-700 pounds. *Every* single very large person with whom I have worked, has dieted repeatedly and consistently throughout his or her life. Dieting and food restriction are the most likely way to increase your weight over the long term!

Weight change and weight stabilization are NOT simple matters. Clearly there are more mechanisms at work here than just the individuals ability to guess calorie consumption and energy expenditure. ***Science does not understand the complicated weight maintenance mechanism.*** That is why, at this time, there is NO medication that can promise more than a 5% to 10% loss in body weight. There is NO pill that results in permanent weight loss. That is why EVERY single weight loss program has a failure rate of over 90%. (That is, over 90% of those who lose weight, gain in back within 5 years.)

Even The Weight Loss Registry from The University of Pittsburgh Medical Center helps to demonstrate this fact. The Registry was started in 1993. The media often uses the people in The Registry as proof that weight loss is a simple matter of calorie control. I would like you to consider the following statistics before you believe the media hype. Can you imagine how many millions and millions of people have lost weight in the nine years between 1993 and 2001? Well, in 2001 there were only 3000 people with "successful" weight loss stories in The Registry. And these are people who have maintained their weight loss for only ONE YEAR! Instead of demonstrating that permanent weight loss is a reasonable expectation for the majority of people, the small number of people in The Registry suggests that the estimate of over 90% failure rate for permanent weight loss is likely to be true.

If science had figured out HOW to lose weight and keep it off, there would be a weight loss pill or program that worked for more than a few individuals. Have you ever seen permanent weight loss statistics released by the various weight loss companies? NO. This information is not released. If science could deliver on the promise of permanent weight loss, weight loss companies would not be refusing to disclose their meager statistics on permanent weight loss.

It is not as simple as we have been told. Science does not, at this time, have the power to control body weight. If you ignore this FACT, and choose weight loss as a primary goal, then you will likely be among the casualties of the diet wars (over 90% failure rate at long-term permanent weight loss.) If you encourage others to choose weight loss as a primary goal, then you are encouraging them to climb onto the weight-loss, weight-gain merry-go-round.

When you consider the fact that we do not, at this time, have the power to control body weight, then what goal can you strive toward? What goal can you recommend to others? You need achievable goals, goals at which you CAN succeed.

1.) **Focus on the ACTIONS of healthy eating.**
2.) **Focus on the ACTIONS of regular exercise and overcoming the obstacles to exercise.**
3.) **Focus on the ACTIONS that meet your emotional needs.**
4.) **Focus on the ACTIONS that improve your relationships.**
5.) **Focus on the ACTIONS that improve your environment.**

Please do not hurt yourself with the ineffective goal of weight loss. Please do not hurt other people by recommending this disappointing goal to others. DO NOT focus on weight loss as a primary goal. Do not teach your children, friends, students, clients or patients to focus on weight loss as a primary goal.

Focus on the ACTIONS of healthy living as your primary goal. Whatever happens with your weight is not under your control. Whatever happens with your weight is a side effect of your healthy living actions.

Watching your weight is an ANXIETY
NOT an action[TM]**.**

Do not focus on weight loss as a primary goal.

Whatever happens with your weight
is a side effect of your actions,
not a goal.

You may not have control over body weight, but you DO have the power to affect your lifestyle. You can get moving, enjoy healthy foods, and cope with emotions without always using food.

When you separate these healthy-living goals
from weight loss,
you will have goals that are achievable!

I have never seen a client damage their self-esteem by adding reasonable, enjoyable exercise to their lives. I have never seen harmful side effects from eating healthier foods. I have never seen eating disorders result from learning to meet emotional needs more effectively. These are constructive goals. These goals don't hurt! When we focus on lifestyle goals (without weight loss expectations or requirements) we have chosen goals that CAN be achieved. I often say to my clients:

"It does not matter what you weigh.
It matters how you live!
Does your life meet your needs?"

Give Yourself a POP

All things in nature change slowly and in cycles. Winter gradually gives way to spring. One day it is warm and balmy. It feels like Spring has arrived. It seems like the seasons are really progressing. Then, out of the blue, the next day it is cold and bitter. When this happens, it can feel like Spring will never arrive. But you know better. You have been through so many changes of the seasons that you have faith in the progression of the seasons. Even if the weather cycles from spring-like days back to cold winter days, you KNOW Spring is coming.

You can build that same faith in your ability to make positive changes in your lifestyle. One action at a time, you will experience yourself going back to healthy living, even after a set back. As you experience your own positive choices, you can build your FAITH in your progress over time. Just as surely as winter turns to spring, you can and will make healthier choices over time. With two steps forward and one step back, you will feel yourself gradually making progress. There are three things necessary for this process to unfold in your life: Persistence, Opportunity, and Patience, (one of my clients called this threesome **"POP"**.)

Persistence

Keep at it. Understanding the cyclical nature of change is important. When you do something helpful to your healthy living, appreciate yourself and your accomplishment. When you do something that you regret ... LEARN from your mistakes. Don't beat yourself up with guilt. Back up. Think about what led to your mistake. Understand what you needed that was missing, or what was too much. Back up and solve the problem that contributed to the mistake. Be persistent. Successes are wonderful. You will also experience setbacks, errors, and mistakes. Every one of these problems is another chance to learn about yourself and your life. Be persistent and keep solving the problems that get in the way of progress. All things in nature change. You can change for the better if you are persistent.

Opportunity

Give yourself the opportunity to improve. Give yourself the chance to learn how to make better choices in your life. Write in your journal, read books, take classes, watch programs that help, talk to helping professionals, talk to helpful friends, etc. Expose yourself to the opportunity to LEARN new ways to cope with old problems.

Often the pain we know seems easier to cope with than the unknown, even if the unknown may be less painful. That is an illusion. Familiarity with pain does not make it comfortable. Even with the scary nature of change and growth, it is worth it. Give yourself the opportunity to grow and learn. You deserve it.

Patience

Positive change sometimes comes like a bolt of lightning. It really feels good when that happens. But more often it creeps in slowly, in cycles forward and back. That is why I suggest that you make positive changes that feel good. If you are enjoying yourself as you change, even if the change is slow, who cares? You are having an enjoyable time anyway. It is easier to be patient.

For example, let's say you really want more physical stamina. You want to be able to do more without being out of breath and without sore muscles. If you choose walking through a beautiful neighborhood or park as your method of building stamina, you are likely to enjoy your process of change. Your motivation can be the pleasure of the walks or the relaxing feeling you get when you let go of all your worries and focus on the flowers around you. Even your goal of achieving more physical stamina is enjoyable motivation (non-critical.)

When you are doing something enjoyable with constructive goals, it is easier to be patient. Change is slow. But if you are enjoying yourself anyway, what do you care if it takes a while before you can feel the changes? Be patient with yourself as you work toward your healthy living goals. Enjoy yourself and how you live. Enjoying yourself helps you to be more patient.

Obstacles or Opportunities
(A True Story In My Life)

I cannot imagine what the ambulance technicians must have thought. They were taking me to the hospital after the car accident. There I was, a thirty-seven year old fat woman in pink spandex tights mumbling, "Oh, no, my body can not be hurt. I make my living with my body!"

I was on my way to a business meeting when the accident occurred. I was to meet my partner to discuss the opening of our new fitness studio in Center City Philadelphia. We were a perfect pair of instructors. She was tall and lean. She looked like the typical picture of an aerobic instructor. I was short and very fit. I was also fat. Between the two of us, all of our clients could identify with an instructor who was similar to them.

It turned out that my body would be fine in a few months. I wish the same were true for my brain. I had a head injury in the accident that resulted in uncontrolled epileptic seizures. I became depressed as I saw my dream go down the drain. What could I do?

I never knew when a seizure would hit. At any moment I could find myself staring into space, not able to understand anything that was said to me, not able to speak, seeing the world through distorted perceptions. For hours afterwards, I could not think. Often I did not even know where I was. How could I live like this? I certainly could not function as a businesswoman. I could not lead my fitness classes. What if I had a seizure in front of the class?

After many months of feeling as if an invisible giant who could knock me senseless at any time was beating me up, I got angry. I decided that I would not let this disability take my life away. After all, I was a trained psychotherapist. I should be able to use the same problem-solving that I taught to my clients to figure out how to live with epilepsy and function in my daily life.

I began to use problem-solving in my own life. When I set my hand on the stove burner during the disorientation that follows a seizure, I found microwave recipes so I could cook safely. When I tried to exercise by walking, I got lost in my own neighborhood. So I walked around my yard instead (I got lost there too, but I found my way home faster.)

I needed to eat well, reduce stress, and get my regular exercise, if I was to fight off depression and cope with my disability. I needed to get my life back. My family shared many of my responsibilities to reduce my stress. I gave extra attention to my nutrition. But exercise remained a challenge.

The reason I began my own fitness company was that I was unable to find any health club, exercise video, or aerobic class that was safe on the joints and was free of size-prejudice. The workout that I had designed was the best workout for me. However, my thinking was impaired from the medications or the seizures or both. I could not remember the moves when I tried to exercise. Then, I got an idea!

I used my home video camera on a tripod to record my workout. I sat down and designed my exercises. Then, I wrote the moves down on a poster board and hung it under the camera. I did not have to remember the moves. They were hanging right in front of me. If I had a seizure, I could turn the camera off for a few hours until I could think better. This was the answer!

I was able to maintain and increase my fitness using a set of my own workout videos. Friends and family who saw my tapes asked me to design a workout and make a fitness video for them. Former clients who missed my unique classes wanted workout videos. Could there be a market for this service? Do I have the ability to do this between seizures?

I sat down and figured out what would be necessary to accomplish this. I had to be more functional. I had to learn to think all over again. I could no longer remember any sequence of ideas or tasks. (As it turns out, I still cannot remember sequences. But I sure got good at conceptual thinking!) It would take time to find the right medications to reduce or control my seizures. During that time I could work on the skills necessary to succeed.

It took three years to find a medication with livable side effects that reduced seizures. During that time, I became computer literate and learned to design and print out advertising materials. I also developed a catalogue of moves I had used in my thirteen years as a full-figured fitness instructor. I did test marketing for my services. Yes, there is a market for custom-made exercise videos that focus on fitness rather than on the shape or size of the body. And yes, I am able to do this!

After the accident, I thought my dream of helping people of all sizes to lead healthier lives was dead. At first, I thought my disability was an insurmountable obstacle that I could not overcome. Well, I did not overcome it. I embraced it. *My head injury was the best educational experience I have had since graduate school!*

The entire idea of making fitness videos to meet individual needs, came from making one to meet my own needs. Through the use of problem-solving, I found an opportunity to make a living because of the way I coped with the obstacles in my life.

If life has cluttered your path with obstacles, you can find opportunities to learn more about yourself and your environment. When you feel overwhelmed, talk to someone who can help. As you use problem-solving to explore your life, who knows what creative solutions lie within yourself waiting to be discovered?

Wake Up Today and Ask ...

Your first thoughts in your day are important. Perhaps you have never noticed what it is, but you do think about something. Notice. Your first thoughts of the day matter. What you think about as you start your day is important. It can set the tone for your day. It can affect your success. I have some suggestions for questions that you might ask yourself upon awakening:

"What did I accomplish yesterday to be helpful?"
or
"What did I do yesterday that made me proud?"
or
"What did I do yesterday to make me be a better person?"

You choose the question that suits you. Make up your own that work for you. The idea is to start your day out with a SUCCESS on your mind. This is a small mental exercise. It may just help. Consciousness helps. Cultivate your appreciation of your positive actions. Start your day off with a question that increases your awareness of your success. **When you are conscious of your success from yesterday, you are already on a positive track for today.** Appreciate your successes from yesterday and you have planted the seeds for your successes today.

Questions and Kelly's Answers

In the first three chapters we looked at "A Fresh Way of Thinking", "Making Peace with Food", and "Fitness and Motivation". In the last chapter we have been playing with "Putting It All Together". Next, I share some "Questions and Answers" so that you can see these concepts as they apply to real life situations.

In this section some of the questions are sometimes from people who cannot imagine separating weight loss from healthy living. You may even hear your own doubts and questions. Notice that in my response, I do not participate in negative assumptions or reinforce them. I simply focus on the positive actions of healthy living.

Whether you are an individual working on self-care or a helping professional trying to learn how to answer questions from your clients and students, this section will be helpful to you. Answering weight loss questions with a non-diet response can be a challenge. You can experience HOW to answer these kinds of questions as you read along. You can imagine how you might answer the questions in your own mind.

You will notice that I use the concepts and phrasing from many other sections of this book as I answer these questions. That is valuable. By using the concepts and phrasing as I answer real world questions, you can more readily imagine how you might answer your students questions or even your own.

Dear Kelly,
Everywhere I turn I see another low carbohydrate diet promising to make me thin. I remember those diets when I was in high school 30 years ago. Back then it just became another part of my yo-yo dieting. Is there something new going on now? Should I give it a try again?

Thanks,
Still Here

Dear Still Here,

I encourage you to listen to the expert on your body. There is only one true expert. That is YOU. If you want to know how carbohydrates affect you, try eating some low carbohydrate meals and notice how you feel. Pay attention to your energy levels, your cravings, and when you get hungry again. Then, on another day, try eating meals and snacks with more carbohydrate content. Pay attention to the same things. You will learn very much from this increased awareness of how food affects you. Choose to eat the foods that make you FEEL best and have the least wrestling with cravings.

I would like you to try something. Experiment with getting more of your carbohydrates from fruits and vegetables. Then notice how you feel. Many people get more energy and more stable blood sugar levels when they enjoy fruits and vegetables as a substantial part of their carbohydrates. You can experiment and see if that is true for you.

I don't know how eating low carbohydrates will feel for you … but your body does know. Trust the expert (you and your body) and listen to what the real expert has to tell you.

Next, and most importantly, if you modify your eating in order to get thin or lose weight, then you are participating in body-criticism. This negative motivation will likely prevent you from maintaining the motivation for long term healthy eating.

I encourage you to eat healthy because your body deserves to feel good. Focus on taking care of the body you have, instead of rejecting your body. In the long run, you will be more likely to build your healthy lifestyle and feel better about your body.

Take care,
Kelly

******

Hi Kelly,
Can you recommend a 30-minute aerobics video for an obese 50 year old to use on those days I don't have time to go to the gym?
Thanks,
Anonymous

Hello Anonymous,
I can tell you what to look for in a workout video so that you will:
- be more likely to use it consistently
- keep you safe when using it
- experience improved fitness as a result of using it

Choose a workout with a focus on fitness and health. Avoid body-critical workouts that promise to make you "look better" or get "a whole new you".

Choose an instructor with a pleasant voice and music that you enjoy. Only high budget videos can afford to get license to use actual artists and original hits. Most workout videos use generic music ... but some is better than others.

Watch for instructors who CONSTANTLY give safety information. You need to know how to do the moves correctly and what common dangerous mistakes to avoid. Find a LOW or NO impact workout for joint safety.

You want to feel successful the first time you do the workout and continue to feel challenged after you have used the video for a while. The instructor MUST show several different ways to do each move so that you can choose the intensity that works for you. Beware of instructors who just say, "tone it down if you need to". The instructor should show HOW to change the moves to meet your needs and still be effective.

You can rent videos at libraries, watch them at video stores, and order videos with a guarantee so that you can return them if they do not meet your needs.

I cannot say for sure if any other workout videos have these important characteristics. Please check some out for yourself. I do know that the many workout videos available at on **www.KellyBliss.com** and **www.PlusSizeYellowPages.com** can be very helpful.

Take care,
Kelly

******

Hi Kelly,
I have joined a weight loss program and have lost 47 lbs. What I need to do now is firm up. I am starting to sag and bag! What are the best exercises for me? I already walk 2 miles and day and work out on exercise machines. My legs and abs really need it.
Thanks,
Annie

Hello Annie,

If you are eating healthy and working out regularly, GOOD FOR YOU!!!! Those are things that you can do for your wellness and health. I hope that you can continue to focus on the healthy lifestyle choices that are good for you.

Studies have shown that the people who appreciate and accept their bodies are the ones who are most likely to continue healthy habits for a lifetime. If you criticize the shape, texture, or size of your body, you will reduce your motivation to take care of yourself. So, right now, what you need to do is make peace with your body and appreciate it.

In answer to your question, "What are the best exercises for you?" You are already doing one of the best exercises you could possibly do... walking. Keep walking. Don't walk to change your body. That would be self-critical. Instead, walk because you deserve the benefits of walking. That is self-nurturing.

Working on various weight machines will improve muscle tone. This may effect the texture of your skin, but that is not the reason to strive for good muscle tone. The reason to work toward strong and flexible muscles is so you can live your life and FEEL good.

I will encourage you to develop ways to think and speak about your body that are less critical. This will really help your feeling of success. There are a few things you can do to take good care of your skin and the softness on your body.

Whenever you walk, wear supportive undergarments on any area of your body that "bounces" or "jiggles". When you support these areas, the collagen elastic fibers in the skin and substructure are not damaged by the bouncing action of walking.

For women, wear a supportive bra to support your breasts. For both guys and gals, a spandex t-shirt will support upper arms, chest, and midriff. For your lower body, guys and gals can wear spandex leggings to support the belly, butt, and legs. The slipperiness of spandex will help with chaffing in the upper thigh area too. You can always wear sweats, T-shirts, or pants on top of these supportive garments if you want.

Feed your body healthy foods that you enjoy.
Exercise regularly for wellness (not body shaping).
Give your body support where it is needed.
Learn to love yourself, body and soul.

Take care,
Kelly

******

Dear Kelly,
I was wondering if you could help me. I am currently in a no-impact aerobics class which I love so very much! However, there are days when I get pressure in my arms due to lactic acid. Can you suggest something for me to do so that I may relieve this? Thank you !
Mary

Hello Mary,
I am impressed. It is difficult to find a no-impact aerobics class and you accomplished it. Congratulations. It is always safest to recommend that you check with your doctor on this matter. He or

she may have some medical advice that would be valuable.

It is likely that the discomfort you are feeling is due to overuse of the muscles in your shoulder and arms. I am guessing that when you say you have "pressure in my arms due to lactic acid", you are referring to that "burning" sensation that muscles get when overused. If this is true, there are several things you can do:

1. Warm-up thoroughly BEFORE you start to lift your arms in the workout. You may want to do some warm-up moves even before the class starts so that you have a few extra minutes for your body to prepare for more intense exercise. This will dilate the blood vessels in your body so that you get more oxygen to the muscles. When you have more oxygen, you will have less build up of lactic acid.

2. Instead of lifting your hands over your head, lift them up slightly in front of your forehead. This puts less strain on the shoulder muscles and is safer for the shoulder joint.

3. Change how high you choose to lift your arms. Just because the instructor has her/his arms up high, does not mean that you should follow. Listen to the real expert... There is really only one expert on your body in the room... That is YOU! When your arms feel fatigue, lower them slightly. After the muscles in your arms and shoulders recuperate, then you can lift your arms up again. Keep listening to your body and keep adjusting to make your workout better for you.

Enjoy! Working out should feel good!
Take care,
Kelly

******

Dear Kelly,
Hi! I have been doing Tae-Bo^{TM} for about a year. I am now doing the advanced class. My problem area is my thighs and buttocks. It seems like my butt is getting bigger, and the cellulite is not going away. I am 5'2" and weigh about 130 pounds. I would like to get toned and am having a hard time. Any suggestions? Thanks,

Regular Exerciser

Dear Exerciser,
I encourage you to pay attention to your lifestyle. Keep working out! Make it fun! Focus on eating enough of the healthy foods, like fruits, veggies, and whole grains. When you are successful at these lifestyle choices, celebrate your success. Appreciate your body for the miracle that it is.

Because you workout vigorously and regularly, by definition, YOU ARE TONED! (even if genetically you are predisposed to have some softness on top of your toned muscles) You cannot judge your fitness and health by the size or texture of your butt and thighs.

Keep taking care of yourself. Buy clothes and exercise wear that support your body and feel good. DO NOT continue to seek an "ideal" body shape and texture. That may cause you to become frustrated and give up on exercising.

It sounds like you do a vigorous workout on a regular basis. That is good. I will caution you to listen to your body. If you become aware of ANY discomfort in your knees, hips, shoulders, or elbows ... DO

NOT IGNORE IT! Tae-bo^{TM} can cause joint problems in many people. If you do develop a problem, there are other ways to get a good workout without joint damage. If you feel no discomfort and want to continue with Tae-bo^{TM}, just keep listening to your body.

Bottom line: Learn to accept your bottom, it is the only one you've got! Keep taking care of yourself, and appreciate your efforts!
Take care,
Kelly

******

Dear Kelly,
I'm Tina and I'm 17 years old. I've had problems with weight since I was 12. I never had problems with weight before age 12. I'm 174 cm tall (5'7") and 80kg (178 lbs.). I have tried to lose weight many times but I was unable to lose a lot of weight. Last year I tried using fitness with a personal trainer but I lost only 6kg (13 lbs.) in four months. Then I gained back 10kg (22 lbs.)!!

I was depressed and very angry. My mother is a psychologist an she was a great support, but still...In December my family and I received news from my doctor's office. She said that the problem is not in "my head".

The problem is that I have too much testosterone in my blood. I'm on medication now but the kg are still here. I eat healthy and I started training for badminton (2 weeks now) but I want my body to look as perfect as possible. I'm young and I just LOVE sports. Do you have any advice for me.

Thank you very much.
Tina

Dear Tina,
Right now you are working on your fitness and your healthy eating. KEEP IT UP! Those are things that you do have control over. Right now you are actively taking care of your medical needs and taking the medication your doctor prescribed. GOOD! This helps you manage your medical problem instead of being the victim of it.

It sounds to me like your body and your weight changed with puberty. That makes sense if your have a testosterone imbalance. I hear the frustration in your message. I also hear something in your message that will make your frustration MUCH WORSE. You say, "but I want my body to look as perfect as possible." Wanting perfection IS a problem. If you want perfection, you will never be satisfied. Seeking perfection causes body loathing, depression, and more.

If you equate thinness with perfection, then you are participating in eating disordered thinking. This is dangerous for your health. Expand your concept of beauty to include a variety of body sizes - including your own. This will help you feel better about yourself. Feeling better about yourself is the most likely way to CONTINUE YOUR HEALTHY LIVING FOR YOUR LIFETIME.

Keep living healthy. Keep active and exercising. Keep eating healthy foods. These are things over which you DO have control. Your weight is a side effect of your individual body, genetics, medical history, diet history, etc. You do not have control over your weight. I recommend that you strive to live healthy and focus on your lifestyle instead of your weight. Your weight will stabilize at the weight that is right for your individual body.

If what I say seems impossible, get support for your journey to self-acceptance. If you are afraid to let go of the ideal of a "perfect" body, seek out support groups, read books that help reduce body-loathing.

Send me your email address and I will make sure to add you as a member of my website. Then you will get my eNewsletter for self-care and self-acceptance. You will find LOTS of resources for your journey to self-care and self-acceptance at www.KellyBliss.com

Take care,
Kelly

******

Dear Kelly,
I started to train few months ago. The first few times I saw the results - they were excellent. I'm overweight. I didn't lose many pounds, but I got my body into shape. Now I have another situation. I still am in shape, but my body size is increasing. My muscles are growing too fast. That's not so nice, because I want to be smaller, not bigger. Will you kindly tell me, what is my mistake? Thank you,
Anna

Dear Anna,
I am so glad that you enjoy fitness training. I hope you are experiencing positive results like improved stamina, flexibility, and strength.

It is unusual for a woman to experience substantial muscle growth. There could be a few things that would contribute to this. You may just naturally have more testosterone than average. This will allow your body to "muscle up". You may be using heavy weights with few repetitions. That is another way to encourage muscle development.

Here are my recommendations. If you want to keep fit and minimize muscle growth:
1.) Include aerobic exercise in your training
2.) Make sure you stretch well after your workout
3.) When using weights, choose LOW weights and more reps.
4.) Keep exercising, no matter what is does to your body size. Moving and exercise are necessary for the human body to function.

I encourage you to exercise for your health and wellness, not to attain some "ideal" body size or shape. Expand your idea of what is beautiful to include a variety of body sizes and shapes, especially your own! This change of mind is not easy. It is worth the effort. By appreciating your own body's size and shape, you are more likely to maintain your healthy living activities.

If you exercise because it FEELS good and it is good for you, then you are more likely to keep exercising as a lifelong habit. Keep moving!

Take care,
Kelly

******

Dear Kelly,
Recently I have had terrible foot pain. I'm told I have
plantar fasciitis, or an inflammation of the bottom of
the foot. Ice and anti-inflammatory (e.g. ibuprofen)
did not do the trick, and the podiatrist I've been sent
to has given me a cortisone shot, told me to stretch
and always wear high heels (it reduces the stretch of
the fascia). My question for you is: how am I
supposed to do your videotaped exercise workout?
Should I try to do it in heels? Should I just keep my
feet flat on the floor? I tried it a little bit, but I didn't
seem to get much of a workout. Any suggestions?
Mimi

Dear Mimi,
First of all, please consult your doctor on medical
problems like this. Next, I may have some useful
information that you can use in your discussion with
your doctor. These are my thoughts as a fitness
professional. Your doctor's advice is what you should
follow.

Think of the arch of your foot like the suspension on
a car. The tendons and ligaments in the arch are like
the springs in a car. When these get overused or over
stretched, you get pain and inflammation. To reduce
the discomfort and allow healing, reduce the overuse
and over stretching.

1. Minimize your walking. (I know, this is difficult to
do with a busy life. Just try.)
2. When sitting, prop your feet up and wiggle your
toes. This will encourage circulation of blood,
synovial fluid (in joints), and interstitial fluid (the
stuff that the lymph system pumps away and cleans).
This gives your tendons and ligaments the best
environment in which to heal.

3. When sitting and you can't prop your feet up, set them on a cool water bottle, well, actually you might want to use two cool water bottles. If it were ice cold, you would not stay there as long because it would be too cold. If it is cool, ahhh, you can enjoy resting the arch of your foot there! This will reduce inflammation.

4. Wear shoes that have a SLIGHT heel, like sneakers that have a nice size heel. Then add a soft arch support with a bit of a heel lift. (You can get these at most drug stores.) This supports your foot, takes the stress off of the tendons and ligaments in the arch.

5. I know the doctor said to take anti-inflammatory. Talk with your doctor about this. I have found that if you only take the anti-inflammatory SOME of the time, you will get little long-term relief. The inflammation comes back between doses. My doctor told me to KEEP anti- inflammatory in my system round the clock for a few days to a week. This breaks the cycle of inflammation. See what your doctor says.

6. When your symptoms subside, EXERCISE. But, exercise in a way that does not irritate or overuse your arches. Do you have some my "Fitness with Bliss^{TM}" video workouts? If you do, that will be a great safe workout if you do one thing ... TAKE THE BOUNCE OUT. I know this is a non-impact workout already. However, I see people in my classes who bounce even though they are not actually jumping. When you take ALL the bounce out and move smoothly with your legs, your arches will be pampered. If you want more aerobic work, add small wrist or hand weights with extra smooth upper body moves as well.

Lastly, be patient. This is an injury that should improve with these steps in a few weeks. However it takes months to completely recover.

Take care,
Kelly

******

Dear Kelly,
I have been exercising (aerobics, stairmaster, etc.) for the last year now, sometimes twice a day. I have lost 20lbs, not enough!!!! I know what my problem is - I do not eat healthy. My question to you is: How do I eat healthy without dieting? I do not like foods with the fancy names. I like to keep it simple: chicken, beef (occasionally), rice, vegetables, green salads and SWEETS! I want to do better.

How many grams of calories and fats should I consume per day to lose weight? Also, I do not understand the nutrition labels on foods. There are total fat, saturated. fat, cholesterol, sugars. You know the label. How much of each should I consume per day?

I am more serious now about my weight. I have to lose 60 lbs for my doctor to consider taking me off my blood pressure medication. Please help.
Shirley

Dear Shirley,
I would encourage you to be more serious about your HEALTHY LIVING and take the focus off of weight loss. This will give you the best chance of continuing your healthy lifestyle.

Be patient. Take the focus off of your weight and soak up your success at exercising. Continue to work on healthy eating. Measure your success by your healthy LIVING, not by your weight. If you focus on your weight, you will get frustrated and give up. If you focus on your successes, you will stay motivated and change for a lifetime.

Keep exercising. Keep eating nutritious foods. For some thoughts on coping with cravings, please check out the section in Chapter Two of this book called: **First, Eat Something Healthy**

Take care,
Kelly

******

Dear Kelly,
I'm 15 years old and way 135lbs I'm also only 5'2. If so, what can I do to lose those extra lbs.
Thanks,
Tubby teen

Dear Teen,
I encourage you to work on building your healthy lifestyle. Gradually work your way up to eating more fruits and vegetables, until you are eating 5 to 8 servings a day. (That will take a lot of focus and attention to accomplish that goal. It is worth it. It will improve your health.)

Increase your activity and exercise in ways that you enjoy. Work toward exercising 4 to 6 days a week. Include some aerobic activity, some muscle toning, and some stretching. This goal will take your attention and your energy as well. Good.

I encourage you to put all your attention on your healthy lifestyle. I hope you will measure your success, not on the scale, but rather by looking at your actions. Whatever your size, small or large, when you take care of yourself with healthy eating and regular movement, then you ARE a success. Check out the section on www.KellyBliss.com called "Track Your Success". You CAN succeed at healthy living ACTIONS.

What about your weight? Watching your weight is not an action. IT IS AN ANXIETY.

My recommendation is to stop focusing on weight loss and focus on your healthy lifestyle. Enjoy your success at eating healthy and exercising regularly.

If you focus on your weight, you will probably hop on the weight loss and gain merry-go-round. That causes weight gain. If you want your body to be your best natural weight, instead of an artificially high weight caused by yo-yo dieting, FOCUS ON YOUR LIFE AND NOT YOUR WEIGHT. Learn to love and enjoy your body. It is the only one you've got!

Take care,
Kelly

******

Dear Kelly,
I never did this before so here I go i think or know
I'm over weight and I try to lose it but I don't know
how I'm going to the gym and I don't think it's
helping, I don't eat the hole day for a week and that

does not help not a little . I am 13 and 200-250 pounds and I hate it please help me.
Angle

Dear Angle,
The most important thing I can tell you is to check out all the support and information on www.PlusSizeYellowPages.com and www.KellyBliss.com Subscribe to the eNewsletter by becoming a member. Use your own Online Workbook. Find self-esteem boosting exercise videos and classes. Get what you need to take care of yourself. You ARE worth it! Expose yourself to this new way of looking at self-care and self-acceptance.

You are trying. You are just doing unhelpful things. The following list seems simple. Sometimes it is. Sometimes it is difficult. But these goals are worth your effort because they result in feeling better and being healthier! To do simple things, you need to get creative. Try putting your time and energy into doing these things:

1.) Eat when you are hungry. If you skip meals or go hungry, you are slowing down your metabolism.
2.) Eat healthy foods, like fruits, vegetables, and whole grains. When you fill up on these, you will have less room for junk food.
3.) Enjoy your food, SAVOR IT! If you don't taste what you eat, you will probably eat more so you can feel it.
4.) Stop eating when you are full. (You can always eat again when you get hungry.)
5.) Take a walk TODAY. Even if you can only take a short walk. JUST START.
6.) Find fitness that FEELS GOOD! Find a plus-size fitness facility where you feel comfortable.

Or, you can use exercise videos that are made for plus-size people.

7.) Stay off the scales. Measure your success by noticing your healthy eating and fitness ACTIONS. This will keep you motivated toward self-care.

THESE ARE THE BEST THINGS YOU CAN DO TO FEEL BETTER ABOUT YOUR BODY AND LIVE HEALTHY!

You CAN feel better. I know. I see people do it all the time.

Take Care,
Kelly

******

Kelly Bliss,

I am a 31 year old female who has two children, 3 years old and 7 months old. I just had a rude awakening about my weight when I wanted to go buy a pair of jeans. When my size 14 didn't fit I realized I needed to go to a 16. At that time I made a decision that I was not going to settle with my weight the way it was. I wanted to learn how I can return to my pre-pregnancy weight at 130 lbs. I immediately signed up for a membership at a gym and started about two weeks ago doing aerobics and lifting weights. I also realize that my eating habits were not helping matters either. So I am trying to learn about a healthier way of eating. When should I see some type of results? I am drinking approximately 1 1/2 quarts of water a day I have totally cut out sodas. I am taking approximately 30-40 fat grams a day also I still am nursing my 7-month-old. Can you give me what my ideal day should be as far as what I can eat and still see results. My height is approximately 5'3.

Can't wait to hear from you give me as much advice as you can so I can take it and run.
31 and 130

Dear 31 and 130,
Many of the actions you describe sound like a great part of a healthy lifestyle. I am glad that you are doing aerobics and lifting weights. This can help you feel more physically fit and psychologically able. Drinking enough water so that your body has what it needs will help your body function better. This is all good for you.

I am concerned however, about the REASON you are making these lifestyle changes. If you do all these things because you hate your body the way it is and you want to lose weight, then every thing you do becomes an act of self-criticism.

I have NO idea if or when your body will return to your pre-pregnancy size and shape. That is the result of a complex set of influences: genetics, weight loss and gain history, medications, etc.

I do know that if you learn to love the body you have, you will be more likely to take care of yourself over time. When you take care of yourself over time, then your body FEELS best. Feeling good is a self-sustaining motivation to continue your healthy living actions.

I also know that if you learn self-acceptance and self-care now, you will be able to teach these concepts to your two beautiful children ... what ever size and shape they turn out to be.

Wishing you well,
Kelly Bliss

"With Bliss" is What Matters

I call the process that I teach "Healthy Living with Bliss™". The most important aspect of this concept is "with bliss". If it is not blissful, then you won't continue to do it for a lifetime.

There are those who believe that all motivation can be summed up in two basic categories: pain and pleasure. Pain is a powerful short-term motivator. Pain simply does not work as a long-term motivator. It is depressing and exhausting. Anyone who has suffered the pain of living large in a small world knows this is true. Anyone who has suffered the pain of an eating disorder knows this is true. Pleasure is a great long-term motivator. When you make changes in your life with pleasure, joy, and bliss as your motivator, you can continue those changes for a lifetime.

Positive motivation is self-sustaining.

In order to be successful with your healthy lifestyle choices, those choices must be pleasurable, comfortable, and enjoyable. Indeed, in order to last a lifetime, choices must be blissful.

In this section I would like to give some concrete examples of what it would be like to cope with eating and exercise issues in this new blissful way. I am going to describe a fictitious day in the life of a fictitious woman. Let's call her Mary. In this day, Mary will encounter all sorts of situations around food and fitness. She will demonstrate the process of healthy eating and fitness with bliss. Mary demonstrates making choices, and working through old thought patterns/feelings. You have read the concepts, now let's see some concrete examples of these concepts in use. Mary faces many of the same situations you face. Perhaps she faces more in a day than you do, perhaps less. She copes with these situations without deprivation, without pressuring, and without guilt. Her motivation is pleasure centered. She actually avoids negative motivation because she knows it is short-term and may cause problems. She makes her life choices with bliss.

Yes, this is a fictitious day, an ideal day. This day is has more choices and more experiences in it than an average day. This day seems longer because I am giving many examples of many choices. I tell you about this day to demonstrate these healthy living concepts in context of daily life. All these events don't happen on one day in a real life. Mary would not always cope as well as she does on this ideal day. I am telling you about this fictitious day for a purpose.

As you watch Mary go through her day, you may see thought processes and choices that would be helpful in your life. Good. You can take steps to add these helpful options to your own life. As you watch Mary go through her day, you may see things that don't apply to you. Fine. Toss those ideas aside and keep looking for helpful ideas. You are in charge of keeping what you find useful and tossing what doesn't work for you. As you watch Mary go through her fictitious day, you decide what is right for you.

Mary's Day

Upon awakening:

Mary finds her fitness gear right in front of her as she heads into the bathroom. "Oh, yeah, today I planned to do a morning workout." She might have forgotten, but the piles of fitness clothes right in front of her give her a physical reminder. As soon as she sees those fitness clothes, she realizes that **last night, when she set out her fitness gear, she had already started her workout**. Momentum has already carried her closer to action. Mary would have to change her mind in order to stop her workout. At this point, it is easier to go with the momentum and continue her workout.

Well, on this day, even with her fitness gear all laid out, she's thinking about skipping the workout. She is feeling like not exercising today. She is thinking about changing her mind because she feels too groggy to move. And then it happens. Mary remembers that she DOESN'T have to workout! Long ago she found out that there was a better choice for her. **Instead of making a commitment to workout, she only made a commitment to dressing and warming-up.** Sometimes she just can't make herself workout. But she can almost always make herself just dress and warm-up. That is what she does today.

Mary thinks: "What type of warm-up should I do? What workout would be right for me today?" Sure, some days Mary makes that choice ahead of time: to walk, or do a video, or head to the pool, or go for a bike ride, or go to the morning class you like in the size-accepting fitness center, or stretch and breathe, or whatever. This is not one of those days. Last night Mary did not feel like making a choice. She just put fitness clothes for a couple of options on her dresser and stuck her "Fitness Menu" on top of the center pile.

Now is the time when she will tune in to how she feels and choose which workout is right for her today. **She thinks about it. She feels into it. She can choose ANY workout on her fitness menu.** What is right for her today? Mary likes the freedom. She likes making choices for herself instead of feeling like she is following some outside set of rules. Mary notices that she doesn't have the old resistance she used to have. There is nothing to rebel against. She can choose any way of moving that feels right for her, including just doing a relaxing stretch. She doesn't even have to commit to doing the workout. Mary only committed to dressing and warming-up! She CAN do that.

Some days Mary chooses to workout at lunchtime or at the end of the day. It is nice to have choices. She can choose whatever time of day feels right for her workout. On the days when Mary works out later in the day, she makes sure that she brings the appropriate workout clothes with her if needed.

Today, however, she finds her fitness gear right in front of her as she awakens. **Some days Mary chooses to workout in the morning.** This is one of those days. She dresses and warms-up. As usual, once she warms-up, she feels like working out, so she finishes her workout. Her mind can relax. She doesn't need to fit her workout into her day ... it's already done.

Now Mary feels good, really good. Her body feels more flexible, stronger, and more able to move through her day. If Mary were large, she would be able to move through her day more comfortably after her workout. If she were coping with chronic pain, she would know that she has done the best she can to minimize that pain by gently rhythmically using muscles and joints. If she were trying to improve her body image and reconnect to her body, she would have appreciated how her body moves. That helps. Mary can take her warm flexible worked out body (and her pink cheeks) and move on with the rest of her day.

Breakfast:
The thought passes through Mary's mind briefly, like a wisp of a cloud. "If I skip breakfast, then I can skip all those calories." She recognizes that pathological thought and answers it: "Garbage!" or "old junk I learned that is NOT true!" Then, Mary replaces the hurtful thoughts with constructive concepts. "My body needs and deserves to be fed!" **Mary has found her own phrase to vehemently disagree with hurtful damaging thoughts that she was taught. She is building the skill of positive thinking every time she practices this process.** She answers these negative thoughts quickly, almost as a reflex action. The negative thoughts dissipate like a little cloud, in the sunshine. Mary knows that soon those hurtful thoughts will not even creep into her mind. Until then, she is really, really good at answering them.

For breakfast Mary eats some carbohydrates that she finds tasty. Some days it is oatmeal on a place mat with a flower in front of her, some days it is a tasty whole grain bagel on the subway. Through experimentation and noticing how food affects her, **Mary learned that eating protein helps her breakfast to last longer so that she is less distracted from hunger or cravings. She eats some protein too.** Some days it is a lovely omelet with bright vegetables and even parsley on the plate. Some days it is a hunk of low fat breakfast meat slapped on that bagel.

Mary always focuses on eating more "live" food (that's fruits and vegetables.) She is amazed that her primary focus on food is eating more healthy food. Mary is amazed how working on **eating more healthy food has taken the place of restricting any foods at all.** And now, at breakfast today, Mary is trying to figure out how to add some fruits and/or veggies to her meal. Some days she has a colorful fruit salad that she spent time preparing. Some days she just drinks a glass of real fruit juice.

Mary remembers, almost with a chuckle, when she used to wonder: "what portion size is correct?" Now Mary does not measure portions. Now she knows that measuring portions, or counting points, or monitoring her eating, actually CAUSES her to react to restricted eating. Now she knows that restricted eating CAUSES bingeing and compulsive eating. On this morning, Mary is eating a healthy balanced meal. She in eating as much food as she wants. **Mary decides how much she wants by tuning in to her own level of satisfaction. As soon as she is satisfied, there is no need to keep eating.**

Mary stops eating when she is satisfied. She can always save the rest for later. That is why they make plastic wrap. She does not restrict her food. She does not overeat. There is no reason to do either. **Mary is at peace with food.** It has been a long process. She is surprised to find herself comfortable around food. She didn't suffer to get here. It was not miserable. It surprises Mary to feel so much better while enjoying herself. Now, Mary is at peace with food, and she has a busy day. She is putting her energy into living her day. Her mind is filled with constructive thoughts. **Mary is focused on her life, not on food, not on weight.**

Mid-morning:

Often, around mid-morning, Mary gets hungry. Sometimes she realizes that she skipped the protein in her breakfast and that may be why she is hungry. Sometimes there is no particular reason. She is just stomach growling hungry. Mary remembers when she used to "resist eating between meals". That was part of the many diets in her life. These diets resulted in repeated weight gains over time. Now, when Mary is hungry, she EATS. No more diets. **Mary makes sure she has access to healthy foods, so that whenever she is stomach growling hungry, she can always enjoy something tasty and healthy to eat.**

Having access to healthy food was not a simple task for Mary to accomplish. At first she tended to put herself down when she could not do the simple task of packing a snack or a lunch. Then, she changed her mind. She refused to blame herself, realizing instead that there were good reasons for the difficulties she has experienced. Mary spent weeks (no, it was months) solving many problems and overcoming obstacles to healthy eating. She worked on her schedule in order to be able to shop. She organized her kitchen in order to store food and have portable containers for her healthy foods. She even went out and got a new briefcase so she could carry her insulated lunch bag. **She was surprised at all the little details that went into having access to healthy foods. And now, today, Mary is proud that she accomplished this complicated task.** Because now, this morning, she gets to take her break and have an enjoyable healthy snack. She will not experience wrestling with her conscience, or repression of her appetite, or guilt about eating. Mary can eat when she is hungry. She can stop when she is full. It's no big deal. She has more to think about in her busy day. She has more to do in her life.

Lunchtime:

Mary thinks: "Man, oh man. THIS has been a good day so far. I exercised. I ate my healthy breakfast. I had a good snack. If I keep this up, I can really lose weight. As a matter of fact, if I only eat soup and salad at lunch, I would lose weight faster." Then it hit her. Mary realized that she has been sucked into the "Diet Vortex". She thought about it. She could feel the old pattern of dieting creeping into her thinking. **EVERY time she has focused on weight loss, she has started to deprive herself. EVERY time she has deprived herself, she found herself with a rebound weight GAIN or with increased eating-disordered thinking.**

Mary is surprised that she could be sucked into the diet vortex after so long at this process of healthy eating based on self-acceptance. She is also pleased that she caught herself and can change her mind. Mary reminds herself that deprivation hurts her. She thinks back to all the enjoyment and healthy choices she has made. She knows that she will continue to feel better about her relationship with food, her body, and her life if she steers clear of the diet vortex. **She knows she needs to listen to her internal cues and meet her own needs.** Now, what's for lunch?

Today Mary is eating at a small cafeteria. There is not much selection of healthy food. Mary is hungry. There was a time when this situation would have caused her to skip lunch or to think: "Forget about it … I can't follow the program anyway. I might as well eat all the junk food I can now. Tomorrow I will start over." Now, this situation does not have the torment of "all or nothing" thinking. Mary has learned to make the best choice she can. Mary deserves to be comfortably full, get as much nutrition as she can, and enjoy her lunch. She will choose foods that taste good and are as healthy as possible. Then, she will not worry about it. **She is not on a program. She cannot fall "off the program". It is no big deal. It is only lunch.**

Mid-afternoon:

As Mary pours water from the pitcher on her desk, she remembers when she used to limit her water intake. If Mary drank a lot of water, then she would have to go to the bathroom more often. Back then, she felt like it was an intrusion into her workday. (Back then she also felt bad about her body and wanted to minimize how much she walked around in front of her co-workers.) Also, Mary did not feel entitled to take breaks for something so trivial as going to the bathroom. Then, she thought about her co-workers who smoked. You can bet that the smokers ALWAYS took their breaks. She thought, "If they can take a break to do something unhealthy, then I sure as heck can take a break to do something healthy."

Now, Mary keeps water available at all times. She keeps a pitcher of water on her desk. She stretches her legs and goes to the bathroom whenever needed. (She feels good about her body. It does not matter what she weighs.) She has better energy because she is not dehydrated. She is actually a better worker BECAUSE she takes care of herself.

It was not always this way. Mary had real trouble working out a system that would allow her to have access to water. At first she set the familiar goal, "I will drink eight glasses of water a day." She did not succeed at that goal. **She backed up (instead of beating herself up.)** "What gets in the way of drinking water?" The answer popped into her head: "I hate the taste!" Now, she had a new goal, "I will find some convenient way to improve the taste of my drinking water." By changing her goal, that is, by having dynamic goals, Mary was one step closer to solving the problem. She kept working on the taste of the water with filters, lemon slices, and keeping it VERY cold. **Her dynamic and flexible goals gave her the room to solve this problem.** Now, she has tasty water in a thermos on her desk.

Suppertime:

Tonight Mary is going out to dinner. She's not just going out to the local diner. She is going to a restaurant where people "dress". So, tonight Mary is dressing up. She goes to her closet to find something to wear. She thumbs through a few outfits and selects one. As she is dressing she notices the wonderful progress she has made.

In years past, Mary used to have a closet filled with clothes that were too small. She used to think that having small clothes around would motivate her to lose weight. It never worked. The clothes that did not fit made her feel like SHE did not fit. It was depressing and it made her feel bad. When she felt bad, she did not take good care of herself.

Mary decided she needed to have clothes that fit. She deserved clothes that fit. It was a process. She started with her sock drawer. (This seemed an easier place to start than her closet. She needed to start small.) Mary got rid of anything that did not fit. She filled the sock drawer with socks that did not bind her calf or squeeze her foot. When she opened her sock drawer, she could grab any pair of socks she wanted. They all fit her! She moved on, a little bit at a time, until her dresser was filled with clothes that fit her.

Then she moved to her closet. It was not easy to give up on the fantasy of turning back the hands of time and recapturing her past days. The sparkly jackets from the mid 1980s were just waiting for her to return to the size she was in the mid 1980. Wait a minute. She could only wear those to a 1980 costume party. Not only has Mary changed, but also Mary acknowledges that the fashions have changed. She donates some clothes to a "Dress for Success" program, some to other charities, and some she sold at a consignment store. Mary was moving into the present and leaving the past behind.

As Mary dresses for dinner tonight, she feels good about how she looks. **She likes her clothes and she feels better about her body. This was a process too. Mary had to learn to be open to beauty that looked like her.** She often reads fashion and lifestyle magazines that have photos of beautiful women who resemble her. She has decorated her house with artwork that features beautiful plus-size people. She has learned to see beauty in diversity and individuality.

So now, with her new-found confidence and her clothes that fit, Mary is going out to dinner. She is looking forward to it. She has gained much experience at enjoying her meal when she is eating it, and afterward when she is comfortably full. She will enjoy eating when she is hungry, and she will enjoy stopping eating when she is satisfied. Mary knows she really can "have her cake and eat it too."

Mary uses a technique to make sure she enjoys her food and gets what she truly wants. **She does not look at the menu. Instead, she focuses internally and decides what kind of food she wants. Then, and only then, does she look at the menu.** When Mary already knows what she has a taste for, then she can open the menu and find it. This way, Mary is not diverted or distracted by the photographs of foods or other external stimuli. She can order exactly what she wants.

Evening:

Evening time varies so much from one night to another. On this evening, after eating a nice meal and being comfortably full, Mary does not even think about food later in the evening. In order to get a better picture of how Mary copes with the night-time munchies, it might be most useful to look at three separate evenings that may have occurred in Mary's recent past.

On one particular evening, after dinner Mary had a relaxing evening planned. She was just going to let go of the day's stress and watch a movie. Then it hit her. She wanted popcorn. She wanted it badly. Mary remembered when this situation would have triggered a cascade of mental wrestling: "To eat or not to eat?" This time it was no big deal. Mary decided to have the popcorn, under one condition. She promised herself that she would really enjoy each and every bite. **Since she was only eating it for the enjoyment and pleasure of it, she might as well enjoy it! She did.** Half way through the bowl, she found that the popcorn did not taste as wonderful as it did in the beginning of the bowl. Since it did not taste as good, Mary was done eating. She was satisfied. No guilt, no problem.

On another evening, Mary had arrived home after a really stressful day at work. She ate the frozen dinner she had prepared last weekend. (Thank goodness for those little freezer containers that make cooking ahead so easy and possible.) Even though she was full, Mary wanted something else to eat quite intensely. She ate one food and then another. Mary noticed that this eating was having an effect on her emotionally. It was numbing her. **Then she realized that she was actually anesthetizing herself with food.** She was wrapping herself in a food cocoon to insulate herself from feeling anything.

Once she realized this, she could think of three choices:

1.) She could just continue to use this food cocoon tonight and figure this out tomorrow. After all, thinking and feeling was exactly what she was trying to escape.

2.) She could just stop now, escape into a book or a movie for now, and figure out what was bothering her later.

3.) She could just stop now, and cope with her feelings NOW. She could write in her journal. She could write without structure, without judgment. She could write free flow and just see what comes out. OR she could call her friend and talk this out. Why did she want to numb herself? What was she escaping from? Mary knew she would get closer to knowing if she wrote or talked.

Mary remembered the outcome of choice #1: nausea, heartburn all night, sometimes a headache, and feeling awful the next day. With that awareness, she decided not to continue her food cocoon. She also did not want to think or feel anymore tonight, so she did not choose option #3. Instead, Mary consciously decided to tune out and read a book (It is easier not to eat when turning pages.) That is fine. **Any choice would have been fine. Because it was a conscious choice instead of an automatic reflex, Mary has the option to figure things out now or later.**

With this awareness, it is less likely that she will get wrapped up in the diversion of "to eat or not to eat?" Mary knows this is not about the food, it is about something in her life. **She will not get tangled up in dieting guilt or body loathing. She knows she has something emotional going**

on that needs tending. Mary can choose to tend her emotional needs now or later. Her emotional needs will not go away. Her emotional needs will be there until Mary takes care of them. Since Mary chose to tune out on this particular evening, she also called a friend and set a date to talk about what was bothering her in the near future.

On yet another evening, Mary had the munchies. She couldn't quite decide if she wanted something sweet or salty. As she asked herself that question, she realized it was the wrong question. "What do I really need?" she asked herself. The answer popped into her head … "I need to celebrate that I got through this day!" "I need a reward." At the moment of the munchies, Mary could not think of a single way to meet this need, except by eating something. Wait. Mary remembered making a list of things to do or give herself when she needed a reward. She looked through her "Own Book" and found the page. There were four lists of things to give herself a reward. Each list included activities that took different amounts of time to do. She had the entire evening ahead of her, so she did not choose activities from her "List for Life" that took a few minutes or 15 minutes. She chose something that would take an hour or more, a bubble bath. She really enjoyed her bath. She relaxed and felt like she had given herself an evening at a spa. What a nice reward after her difficult day.

Not Easy

As you read about the fictitious day described here, it may sound too simple. I don't mean to imply that there are no struggles involved in this process. The road to self-acceptance and self-care includes plenty of struggles. It is not easy. It takes time and effort. It is downright difficult at times.

However, this is a road worth traveling **because you CAN succeed at these goals**. Most of the difficulties arise when you veer away from self-acceptance and accidentally slide into self-critical attitudes or behavior. Other troubles arise when you tune out and shut down your awareness leading to self-abusive behavior. In both of these cases, it becomes difficult to take care of yourself. The challenge is to tune in and take care.

The good news is that when you feel pain or start to do hurtful things, you can think of these as RED FLAGS! Once you see a red flag, then you can steer yourself back toward more constructive attitudes and behaviors. More good news is that when you recognize the red flags and take action, you will feel better physically and emotionally. You cannot fail. As soon as you realize that you are participating in self-criticism or destructive behavior, that is when you have the opportunity to change and move back toward self-acceptance and self-care.

Think of someone riding a bike. They do not steer straight center with their arms locked. Instead they veer a little to the right and a little to the left. This swerving right and left a tiny bit IS how a person steers straight toward the center on a bicycle. Your journey will be much the same. Sometimes you will veer off toward self-criticism. Sometimes you will veer off toward tuning out. That's OK. That is part of the process.

What will make your struggle worth the effort? Because at any given moment, once you get used to seeing the red flags and solving the problems, **it FEELS better to take care of yourself! What will motivate you to continue is ENJOYMENT and PLEASURE.**

If I Can Do It, You Can Too.

I read about people who preach weight loss. I hear hysterically energetic gurus of dieting and fitness talk about constant life-long battles with appetites, compulsive eating, and with food. The audience is told by the laughing and crying guru, "I am in the same struggle as you are. I have the same compulsions as you do. I am a compulsive overeater too. I have been my entire life and I always will be. If I can do this, then so can you." Time and time again the weight loss experts say they want you to join them in their struggles. They are fighting the "good fight" against food and appetite. They want you to join them in this battle against the body.

**I am saying something profoundly different to you.
I do NOT want you to join me in a lifelong battle
against food or against your appetite.**

**I want you to find peace with food,
develop an active lifestyle,
appreciate your body,
and get on with living your life
in the body you have!**

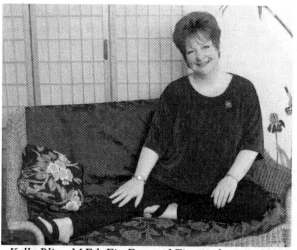

Kelly Bliss, M.Ed, Fit, Fat, and Fine in the year 2000

I invite you to join me in my RECOVERY from body loathing and weight loss anxiety. I invite you to join me in ending compulsive eating instead of controlling it. I do NOT recommend that you fight your appetite. Your appetite is an asset to healthy eating. I do not recommend that you "control your weight." Your weight is the result of many things, some of which are out of your control.

I recommend that you participate in the fun and enjoyable problem-solving process that will help you live your healthy life. How your body changes and responds to your improved healthy lifestyle is not under your control. That is a complicated process that not even the most advanced science has unraveled. Perhaps the way your body changes and responds to your healthy lifestyle is in the hands of something bigger than you. You do have the power to influence your lifestyle and your attitudes. I invite you to join me in influencing your lifestyle and your attitudes.

I am about to tell you a list of statements about myself. I tell you these things because these are the answers to questions that I am often asked by clients who want hope. I tell you these things because I want you to know there is hope. Even though there are many, many people who have made a similar journey, in the following statements I am speaking for myself. I want you to join me in an enjoyable struggle to make peace with yourself. If I can do it, so can you...

    ** I used to be a compulsive overeater.
       Now I am at peace with food.

    ** My appetite used to be my enemy.
       Now my appetite is an asset to healthy eating.

    ** I used to HATE my body.
       Now I appreciate how my body looks, feels, and
       functions. I truly take joy in my physical self.

    ** I used to be very sedentary for long periods of time.
       Now I really ENJOY workouts regularly.

** I used to abuse my body, running three hours per day. Now I workout gently and reasonably.

It has been a long struggle for me to heal from dieting and the body-loathing that dieting cultivates. It has taken great effort to recover and get to this point. This struggle and effort were enjoyable! During my struggle, every few months I would look back and notice how much BETTER I was feeling. This struggle was self-motivating.

Yes, I invite you to join me in this enjoyable struggle to take care of yourself. If I can do it, you can too. You can respond to feeling better as you make choices with awareness.

**You can accept yourself, care for yourself,
and enjoy living your life.**

**This is a long, enjoyable process.
It feels good.**

**I invite you to feel good.
You deserve it!**

Appendix I

Current Resources

You will find a complete up to date list of current resources for living large in a small world at www.PlusSizeYellowPages.com There are over 2000 listings for everything you need to live large in a small world. If you are not hooked up to the Internet, you can always log on at your local library. Below is the list of some of the categories listed in Kelly Bliss' Plus Size Yellow Pages™:

Body Image	Health	Personal Care
Books	Professionals	Pets and Hobbies
Bridal	Home Furnishings	Plus Size Art
Catalogs	Jewelry and	Plus Size Kids
Clothing: Children	Accessories	Plus Size Modeling
Clothing: Juniors	Legal	Sew Your Own
Clothing: Men	Professionals	Size Friendly
Clothing: Women	Legal Resources	Travel
Costumes	Lingerie	Sporting Goods
Custom Made	Magazines	Sportswear
Eating Disorders	Maternity	Swimwear
Fitness	Newsletters	T-Shirts
Footwear	Non-Diet	Uniforms
For People with	Programs	Used-Consignment
Disabilities	Office Furniture	Videos
Formalwear	and Supplies	Wholesale
Health	Organizations	

Appendix II

Magazines

Note: see www.PlusSizeYellowPages.com for most recent list.

BBW (Big Beautiful Woman)
P. O. Box 1297
Elk Grove CA 95818
1-800-877-5549
http://www.bbwmagazine.com/

Belle
475 Park Avenue South
New York NY 10016
1-800-877-5549
http://www.bella-mag.com/

Canada WYDE
PO Box 511
99 Dalhousie St
Toronto, Ontario, Canada M5B 2N2.
cdawyde@interlog.com
http://www.interlog.com/~cdawyde/

ExtraHip magazine
6201 W. Sunset Blvd., #94
Hollywood, CA 90028
1-888-Xat-XHIP (1-888-928-9447)
mail@extrahip.com
http://www.extrahip.com/

Fat!So?
Marilyn Wann, Editor
P. O. Box 423114
San Francisco CA 94142-3464
marilyn@fatso.com
http://www.fatso.com

Freesize
C/O SIZE
Suite 147
56 Gloucester Road
Kensington, London, SW7 4UB

Healthy Weight Journal
Frances M. Berg, editor and publisher
402 South 14th Street
Hettinger, ND 58639
800-663-0023 (US and Canada)
hwj@healthyweight.net
http://www.healthyweightnetwork.com/

Mode Magazine
22 East 49th Street
6th floor
New York, NY 10017
1-888-610-6633
modemag@aol.com
http://www.modemag.com/

New Moon
The magazine for girls and their dreams
P.O. Box 3620
Duluth, MN 55803
1-800-381-4743
lindae@newmoon.org
newmoon@newmoon.org

NZ Bella
177 Parnell Rd.
1st Floor
Parnell, Auckland
New Zealand
kmco@bella.co.nz
http://www.bella.co.nz/

oooO Baby Baby
1448 Fullerton Drive
Fairfield Ca 94533
707-643-0506
ldysrches@aol.com
http://www.oooobabybaby.com

Radiance: Online Magazine for Large Women
P. O. Box 30246
Oakland CA 94604
510-482-0680
radmag2@aol.com
http://www.radiancemagazine.com

Appendix III

Videos

These are videos with self-care / self-acceptance themes -- without body critical or body shaping content.

Note: see www.PlusSizeYellowPages.com for most recent list.

Body Trust: Undieting Your Way to Health and Happiness
Dayle Hayes, M.S., R.D.
Productions West
3112 Farnum Street
Billings MT 59102
1-800-321-9499
EatRightMT@aol.com

Fat Chance: the Big Prejudice
by the National Film Board of Canada
NFBC Customer Services D-10
P. O. Box 6100
Station Centre-Ville
Montreal, PQ
Canada H3C 3H5
(US): 1-800-543-3764
(Canada): 800-267-7710

***Fitness with Bliss*™**
Plus Size and Specialty Fitness
Kelly Bliss, M.Ed.
TEN different fitness videos done standing, sitting, and reclining, so that every body can find the right workout for their individual needs.
Toll Free 877-KellyBliss (877-535-5925)
kelly@kellybliss.com
http://www.KellyBliss.com

Gentle Yoga With Naomi
Naomi Judith Offner, MA
P.O. Box 2097
Delmar, CA 92014
1-800-655-6668
Naomi@gentleyoga.com
http://www.gentleyoga.com

Gorgeous
Film Australia
Pty. Ltd.
P. O. Box 46
Lindfield NSW 2070
Australia

In Grand Form
Plus size fitness
Jody Sandler
1-800-296-3077
http://www.ingrandform.com

Killing Us For Our Own Good: Dieting and Medical Misinformation
Dawn Atkins
Body Image Task Force
P. O. Box 360196
Melbourne FL 32936-0196
bitf@yahoo.com
http://home.earthlink.net/~dawn_atkins/bitf.htm

Look Who's Walking
Orchid Leaf Productions
P.O. Box 72,
Flint, MI 48501

Nothing To Lose
by Fat Lip Readers Theatre
P. O. Box 29963
Oakland CA 94604

Tai Chi Chuan
Dawn Fleetwood
Orchid Leaf Productions
P.O. Box 72
Flint, MI 48501
801-235-9864

Yoga for Large People
Mara Nesbitt-Aldrich
P.O. Box 19141
Portland, OR 97280
www.webrox.net/yogavideo

Yoga for Round Bodies,
Linda DeMarco and Genia Pauli Haddon
P.O. Box 265
Suite 200
Scotland, CT 06264
800-793-0666

Appendix IV

Organizations

Organizations that Promote
Self-acceptance / Self-care Philosophy

Note: see www.PlusSizeYellowPages.com for most recent list.

About-Face
P. O. Box 77665
San Francisco CA 94107,
Phone: 415-436-0212
E-mail: info@about-face.org
Web site: http://www.about-face.org/
Questions and satirizes negative images of women in our culture and promotes alternatives through education and action

Abundia
P. O. Box 252
Downers Grove IL 60515
Phone: 708-897-9796
E-mail: Erdman@cdnet.cod.edu
Annual summer retreat for large women

ANRED (Anorexia Nervosa and Related Eating Disorders)
P. O. Box 5102
Eugene OR 97405
Phone: 503-344-1144

Web site: http://www.anred.com
Advocacy and support, educational materials

Big As Texas
P. O. Box 363
Sour Lake TX 77659
Phone: 409-753-3451,
E-mail: BigAsTexas@juno.com
Web site: http://members.tripod.com/bigastexas/
Annual Spring weekend convention with activism workshops
and social events for large people and their friends

Body Image and Health, Inc.
Thea O'Connor
Director
Phone: (03) 9344 2662
Fax: (03) 9344 2390
E-mail: bodyimage@cryptic.rch.unimelb.edu.au
Program encouraging residents of Victoria to accept, enjoy
and nurture their bodies; newsletter and body image kit

Body Image Task Force (BITF)
P. O. Box 360196
Melbourne FL 32936-0196
E-mail: bitf@yahoo.com
Web Site: http://home.earthlink.net/~dawn_atkins/bitf.htm
Political action around body image issues

The Council on Size & Weight Discrimination
Miriam Berg, President
P. O. Box 305
Mt. Marion NY 12456
Phone 914-679-1209
E-mail: Miriam@cswd.org ,
Web Site: http://www.cswd.org/index.htm
Information, referrals, advocacy

Eating Disorder Referral and Information Center
International Eating Disorder Referral Organization
2923 Sandy Pointe, Suite 6
Del Mar, CA 92014-2052
Phone: 858-481-1515
Fax: 858-481-5143
Web site: http://www.edreferral.com
Information about, and treatment resources for, all forms of
eating, exercise, and body image disorders

EDAP (Eating Disorders Awareness & Prevention)
603 Stewart Street, Suite 803
Seattle WA 98101
Phone: 206-382-3587
Fax: 206-292-9890
Web site: http://www.edap.org
Annual Eating Disorders Awareness Week (EDAW), support
material; EDAW held on February 20-27 this year

Healthy Weight Network
Frances M. Berg, MS
402 South 14th Street
Hettinger, ND 58639
Phone:701-567-2646
Fax:701-567-2602
E-mail: fmberg@healthyweight.net
Website: http://www.healthyweight.net/
Obesity research watchdog organization, advocate for healthy
eating and fitness

Hugs International, Inc.
Box 102 A, RR #3
Portage La Prairie, MB
Canada R1N 3A3
Phone: 204-428-3432
Fax: 204-428-5072
E-mail: linda@hugs.com
Web site: http://www.hugs.com/

A support network for getting off the diet roller coaster; Hugs
Club News, material and workshops for teens

ISAA (International Size-Acceptance Association)
P. O. Box 82126
Austin TX 78758
E-mail: Director@size-acceptance.org
Web site: http://www.size-acceptance.org/
Advocacy, activism, chapters, newsletter

Largely Positive, Inc.
Carol Johnson, Director
P. O. Box 17223
Glendale WI 53217
Phone: 414-299-9295 (voicemail)
E-mail: positive@execpc.com
Size-positive support group, educational handouts, On A
Positive Note newsletter, support groups around the US

Largesse, the Network for Size Esteem
E-mail: largesse@eskimo.com
Fax: 707-929-1612
Web site http://www.eskimo.com/~largesse/
Online resources, information and educational handouts

Melpomene Institute for Women's Health Research
1010 University Avenue
St. Paul MN 55104
Phone: 612-642-1951
Events for large women, info packet, newsletter

NAAFA (National Association to Advance Fat Acceptance)
P. O. Box 188620
Sacramento CA 95818
Phone: 916-558-6880
Web site: http://www.naafa.org
Advocacy, support, local chapters; INDD kit

National Center for Overcoming Overeating
Carol Munter and Jane Hirschmann, Directors
P.O. Box 1257
Old Chelsea Station
New York NY 10113-0920
Phone: 212-875-0442
Web site: http://www.overcomingoverating.com/
Anti-diet support group; workshops, educational material,
centers in several areas, e-mail list

NEDIC (National Eating Disorders Centre)
CW1-211/200 Elizabeth Street
Toronto, Ontario
Canada M5G 2C4
Phone: 416-340-4156
E-mail: mbeck@torhosp.toronto.on.ca
Web site: http://www.nedic.on.ca/
Non-dieting support material, workshops; sponsor of EDAW
and INDD

NOLOSE (National Organization for Lesbians of Size)
245 Eighth Avenue #107
New York NY 10011
Phone: 201-843-4629
E-mail: nolose@aol.com
Web site: http://www.breakinc.com/nolose/
Support and advocacy for lesbians of size, annual conference
held in summer; sponsor of INDD

SCAN (Sports, Cardiovascular and Wellness Nutrition)
90 South Cascade Avenue, Suite 1190
Colorado Springs CO 80903
Phone: 719-475-7751
Fax: 719-475-8748
E-mail: SCAN@fleckcorporation.com
Web site: http://www.nutrifit.org/
Professional organization, sponsors annual conference with non-diet workshops and speakers

SIZE (National Size Acceptance Coalition)
Diana Pollard, Director
Suite 147, 56 Gloucester Road
Kensington London
SW7 4UB England
Phone: 0171 700 0509
Fax: 0171 581 9213
E-mail: dwm@premier.co.uk
Sponsor of international size-positive art exhibit; magazine Freesize

Appendix V

Fitness Wear

Companies that provide plus size fitness wear

Note: see www.PlusSizeYellowPages.com for most recent list.

Ad In Apparel
Web site: http://www.adintennis.com/adintennis.asp
Custom designed tennis wear for women of all sizes - Tennis
dresses up to size 3X; tops, panties and other plus size
clothing

All Ashore
7959 Broadway St #404
San Antonio, TX 78209
210-829-7813
Swimwear in sizes 16W-26W

Bathers for Big Girls
http://www1.tpgi.com.au/users/big_girls
Made to measure swimwear for the larger ladies, bust sizes
from 38 inches to 62 inches.

Beautiful Skier
1-800-638-3334
Ski Wear in sizes 16-30.

Big Day at the Beach
909-798-5228
Custom sizing. Good prices.

Big Head Caps
http://www.bigheadcaps.com/
Extra Large Size Adjustable Baseball Caps

Big on Batik
cathy@bigonbatik.com
http://www.bigonbatik.com/bathing_suits.html
Suits up to size 52. Tel: 760-434-3515.

Big Stitches Swimwear
2423 Douglas St.
San Pablo, CA 94806
510-237-3978
Custom made large-size bathing suits.

BY RO!
310-221-0509
byrodesign@aol.com
http://www.plusshop.com/
Sizes to 5X + custom.

Cabela's
http://www.cabelas.com/
Sportswear to size 5X.

Champion Woman
http://www.championjogbra.com/htm/ch_woman/ch_woman.htm
Workout apparel for women sizes 14 to 28.

Danskin Outlet
1-800-288-6749
Fitness wear in sizes to 4X

Elisabeth by Liz Claiborne
http://www.lizclaiborne.com/elisabeth/default.asp
Sportswear designed for the larger woman.

ENELL Sports Bra
http://www.enelltm.com/
ALL sizes! 34B to 52DDD

Greater Salt Lake Clothing Company
801-273-8700
sales@gslcc.com
http://www.gslcc.com/
Plus size fitness wear and large-size ski clothes

Hot Off the Tour
1-800-878-8189
Specializing in golf wear

JC Penney's
PO Box 2021
Milwaukee, WI 53201-2021
1-800-222-6161
http://www.jcpenney.com
Swimsuits up to size 26W.

Junonia for Active Women
The Minnesota Building, Suite 216
46 East Fourth Street
St. Paul, MN 55101
1-800-671-0175
1800junonia@worldnet.att.net
http://www.Junonia.com/
Swimwear (including two piece!) to 6X.

Just Right
30 Tozer Rd.
PO Box 1020
Beverly, MA 01915-0720
1-800-767-6666
Sizes to 26

LizzyWear.Com

lizzywear@aol.com
http://www.lizzywear.com/
Cotton lycra garments

Love Your Peaches
1-888-274-7499
janelle@loveyourpeaches.com
http://www.loveyourpeaches.com/swimsuits.htm
Mix-n-match swimwear to size 36.

Ocean Ray Wetsuits
1-800-645-5554
oceanray@wilmington.net
http://www.oceanray.com/
Wet suits, for people 350 pounds or more.

Oddessy Martial Arts and Medieval Supply Center
1-800-ODDESSY (1-800-633-3779)
info@oddessy.com
http://www.oddessy.com
Large martial arts uniforms

Queen of Hearts, Inc.
19 Merrick Ave.
Merrick, NY 11566
1-888-783-3633
Swimsuits to size 32.

SanDiegoFit.com
http://www.sandiegofit.com/
Exercise wear sizes to 6X.

Sea-Ragz Enterprise Inc
http://www.searagz.com/
"Real Sized" swim wear!

Shore-Fit Sunwear
http://www.obxsunwear.com/

A swimwear boutique 8 to 28.

Swimsuits Just for Us
http://www.swimsuitsjustforus.com/
Designer swimwear for sizes 16 and up.

Sweat It Out
sweatitout@prodigy.net
www.sweatitout.com
Fitness wear sized small to large and very large.

Ulla Popken
1-800-245-8552
http://www.ullapopken.com/
Swimsuits to size 30.

WaterWear
Riverview Mill
Wilton, NH 03086
1-800-321-SUIT (1-800-321-7848)
Aquatic fitness wear, sizes to 28.

Worldware Plus Size Clothing
3181 Packard
Ann Arbor MI. 48108
Rkarle@aol.com
http://ic.net/~karle/ww/page2.htm
Mail order sportswear sizes 2X to 10X.

Zala Design
Box 80018
Minneapolis, MN 55408
612-871-4809
Catalog $2 Leotards up to size 7X.

Appendix VI

Additional Reading

Writings that promote the
Self-Care / Self-Acceptance Philosophy

Note: see www.PlusSizeYellowPages.com for most recent
list.

I have included a HUGE list of books. I have listed so
many books because I want you to know that there is a wealth
of information about how to live large in a small world. I do
not include all of these books to overwhelm you. Please
consider this list like a buffet. You can pick and choose what
you would like to sample. Try out what interests you.
Explore new experiences. Enjoy.

Acolyte, J: *The Big Bang: The Birth of a New Plus-sized
Universe.* Honor the Circle Astrology Expressions, 1999.

Atrens, Dr. Dale M: *Don't Diet.* New York: William Morrow
and Company, Inc., 1988. ISBN: 0688074693.

Beller, Anne Scott: *Fat & Thin: A Natural History of Obesity.*
New York: Farrar, Straus, and Giroux, 1977. ISBN:
0374219648.

Bennett, William and Joel Gurin: *The Dieter's Dilemma:
Eating Less and Weighing More.* New York: Basic Books,
1982. ISBN: 0465016529.

Berg, Frances M: *Afraid to Eat: Children and Teens in Weight Crisis - Health Risks of Weight Loss*. Hettinger: Healthy Weight Journal, 1997. ISBN: 0-918532-55-5.

Berg, Frances M: *Health Risks of Weight Loss*. Hettinger: Healthy Weight Journal, 1995. ISBN: 0918532442.

Blank, Hanne: *Big Big Love*. Emeryville: Greenery Press, 2000. ISBN: 1890159166.

Bliss, Kelly: *Don't Weight: Eat Healthy and Get Moving NOW!*. Work It Out, Inc., 2000. ISBN:

Bordo, Susan: *Unbearable Weight: Feminism, Western Culture & the Body*. Berkeley: University of California Press, 1993. ISBN: 0520079795.

Bovey, Shelley: *The Forbidden Body: Why Being Fat is not a Sin*. London: Pandora Press, 1989 / New York: New York University Press, 1994. ISBN: 0-04-440871-4.

Brown, Catrina and Karin Jasper: *Consuming Passions: Feminist Approaches to Weight Preoccupation and Eating Disorders*. Ontario, Canada: Second Story Press, 1993. ISBN: 0929005422.

Brown, Laura S. and Esther D. Rothblum, Ed.: *Overcoming Fear of Fat: Fat Oppression in Psychotherapy*. Harrington Park Press, 1989. ISBN: 0-918-393-71-X.

Brownmiller, Susan: *Femininity*. New York: Fawcett Columbine, 1984. ISBN: 0449901424.

Brumberg, Joan Jacobs: *Fasting Girls: The History of Anorexia Nervosa*. New York: New American Library, 1989. ISBN: 0452262371.

Bruno, Barbara Altman, Ph.D.: *Worth Your Weight*. Rutledge Books, Inc., 1996. ISBN: 1887750320.

Burke, Delta and Alexis Lipsitz: *Delta Style: Eve Wasn't a Size 6 and Neither Am I*. New York: St. Martin's Press, 1998. ISBN: 0312154542.

Cannon, Geoffrey and Hetty Einzig: *Dieting Makes You Fat.*
New York: Simon and Schuster, 1985. ISBN:
0671530720.

Carlson, Nancy: *I Like Me.* Puffin Books/Penguin Putnam
Books For Young Readers, 1990. ISBN: 0-14-050819-8.

Chapkis, Wendy: *Beauty Secrets: Women and the Politics of
Appearance.* South End Press, 1986. ISBN: 0-89608-280-
2.

Chernin, Kim: *The Hungry Self: Women, Eating, and
Identity.* New York: Times Books, 1985. ISBN: 0-81-
291146-6.

Chernin, Kim: *The Obsession: Reflections on the Tyranny of
Slenderness.* New York: Harper & Row, 1981. ISBN: 0-
06-090967-6.

Christian, Sandy Stewart: *Working With Groups to Explore
Food & Body Connections : Eating Issues, Body Image,
Size Acceptance, Self-Care (Structured Exercises in
Healing).* Whole Person Associates, 1996. ISBN:
1570251053.

Cooper, Charlotte: *Fat and Proud: The Politics of Size.*
Womens Press Ltd., 1999. ISBN: 0-7043-4473-4.

Curtis, Lucy D. L: *Lucy's List " A Comprehensive
Sourcebook for Making Larger Living Easier.* New York:
Warner Books, 1995. ISBN: 0446672831.

Deckert, Barbara: *Sewing for Plus Sizes.* Newtown: Taunton
Press, 1999. ISBN: 1561582840.

Douglas, Susan: *Where The Girls Are: Growing Up Female
with the Mass Media.* New York: Times Books, 1994.
ISBN: 0812922069.

Ehrenreich, Barbara and Dierdre English: *For Her Own
Good: 150 Years of the Experts' Advice to Women.* Garden
City, NY: Anchor Press, 1978. ISBN: 0385126506.

Emme, et al.: *True Beauty : Positive Attitudes and Practical Tips from the World's Leading Plus-Size Model.* New York: G.P. Putnam's Sons, 1996. ISBN: 0399142045.

Epstein, Diane and Kathleen Thompson: *Feeding on Dreams: Why America's Diet Industry Doesn't Work--And What Will Work for You.* New York: Macmillan Publishing Company, 1994. ISBN: 0025361910.

Erdman, Cheri, Ed.D: *Live Large!* HarperCollins, 1996. ISBN 0-06-251345-1.

Erdman, Cheri, Ed.D*: Nothing To Lose: A Guide to Sane Living in a Larger Body.* San Francisco: Harper San Francisco, 1995. ISBN: 0-06-251253-6.

Ernsberger, Paul and Paul Haskew. *Rethinking Obesity: An Alternative View of its Health Implications.* Monograph issue of The Journal of Obesity and Weight Regulation, v. 6 n. 2. Human Services Press, 1987. ISBN: 0898854083.

Estroff, Hara*: Style Is Not a Size: Looking and Feeling Great in the Body You Have.* New York: Bantam Books, 1991. ISBN: 0553352709.

Fallon, Patricia: *Feminist Perspectives on Eating Disorders.* Guilford Press, 1994. ISBN: 0898621801.

Farro, Rita: *Life Is Not A Dress Size.* Radnor: Chilton Book Company, 1996. ISBN: 080198758X.

Foster, Patricia, ed: *Minding the Body: Women Writers on Body and Soul.* New York: Anchor Books, 1995. ISBN: 0-385-47167-X.

Fraser, Laura: *Losing It: America's Obsession With Weight and the Industry That Feeds on It.* New York: Dutton, 1997. ISBN: 0-525-93891-5.

Freedman, Rita: *Beauty Bound.* Lexington, MA: Lexington Books, 1986. ISBN: 0669111414.

Freedman, Rita: *Bodylove: Learning to Like our Looks and Ourselves, A Practical Guide for Women.* New York: Harper & Row, 1989. ISBN: 006016025.

Friedman, Sandra Susan: *When Girls Feel Fat: Helping Girls Through Adolescence.* Toronto, Ontario: HarperCollins, 1998. ISBN: 1552094596.

Gaesser, Glenn A: *Big Fat Lies: The Truth About Your Weight and Your Health.* New York: Fawcett Columbine, 1996. ISBN: 0-449-90941-7. Contact Glenn Gaesser at gag2q@virginia.edu.

Garrison, Terry Nicholetti: *Fed Up! A Woman's Guide to Freedom from the Diet/Weight Prison.* New York: Carroll & Graf Publishers, Inc., 1993. ISBN: 0881849642.

Gilligan, Carol: *In A Different Voice : Psychological Theory and Women's Development.* Cambridge: Harvard University Press, 1993. ISBN: 0674445449.

Goffman, Erving: *Stigma: Notes on The Management of Spoiled Identity.* New York: Simon and Schuster, A Touchstone Book, 1986. ISBN: 0671622447.

Goodman, W. Charisse: *The Invisible Woman: Confronting Weight Prejudice in America.* Gurze Books, 1995. ISBN: 0936077107.

Gossett, Harry: *Fat Chance!.* Alexandria, VA: Independent Hill Press, 1986.

Grosswirth, Marvin: *Fat Pride: A Survival Handbook.* Jarrow Press, Inc., 1971. ISBN: 0912190051.

Hall, Lindsey, ed: *Full Lives: Women Who Have Freed Themselves from Food & Weight Obsession.* Carlsbad, CA: Gurze Designs & Books, 1993. ISBN: 0936077263.

Head, Sandy Summers: *Sizing Up: Fashion, Fitness, and Self-Esteem for Full-Figured Women.* New York: Simon & Schuster, A Fireside Book, 1989. ISBN: 0671675729.

Herman, C. Peter and Janet Polivy: *Breaking the Diet Habit.* New York: Basic Books, 1983. ISBN: 0465007546.

Hesse-Biber, Sharlene: *Am I Thin Enough Yet? : The Cult of Thinness and the Commercialization of Identity.* New York: Oxford University Press, 1996. ISBN: 0195082419.

Higgs, Liz Curtis: *One Size Fits All and Other Fables.* Nashville: Thomas Nelson Publishers, 1993. ISBN: 0840763336.

Hillman, Carolynn: *Love Your Looks: How to Stop Criticizing and Start Appreciating Your Body.* New York: Fireside, 1996. ISBN: 0-684-81138-3.

Hillman, Carolynn: *Recovery of Your Self Esteem : A Guide for Women.* New York: Simon & Schuster, 1992. ISBN: 0-671-73813-5.

Hirschmann, Jane R. and Carol H. Munter: *Overcoming Overeating.* Reading, MA: Addison-Wesley Publishing Company, Inc., 1988. ISBN: 0201122197.

Hirschmann, Jane R. and Carol H. Munter: *When Women Stop Hating Their Bodies.* New York: Fawcett Columbine, 1995. ISBN: 0449906809.

Hirschmann, Jane R. and Lela Zaphiropoulos: *Are You Hungry? A Completely New Approach to Raising Children Free of Food and Weight Problems.* New York: Random House, 1985. ISBN: 0394541464.

Hutchinson, Marcia Germaine: *200 Ways to Love the Body You Have.* Freedom, CA: The Crossing Press, 1999. ISBN: 0-89594-999-7.

Hutchinson, Marcia Germaine: *Transforming Body Image: Learning to Love the Body You Have.* Trumansburg, NY: The Crossing Press, 1985. ISBN: 0-89594-172-4.

Ikeda, Joanne, RD, and Priscilla Naworski, MS: *Am I Fat? Helping Young Children Accept Differences in Body Size.* ETR Associates, 1993. ISBN: 1560710802.

Jasper, Karin: *Are You Too Fat, Ginny?* Is Five Press, 1988. ISBN: 0920934323.

Johnson, Carol: *Self Esteem Comes in All Sizes*. New York: Doubleday, 1995. ISBN: 0385475659.

Johnston, Joni E: *Appearance Obsession: Learning to Love the Way You Look*. Deerfield Beach, FL: Health Communications, Inc., 1994. ISBN: 1558742700.

Kano, Susan: *Making Peace with Food*. New York: HarperCollins, 1989. ISBN: 006096328X.

Kaplan, Jane Rachel, ed: *A Woman's Conflict: The Special Relationship Between Women and Food*. Englewood Cliffs, NJ: Prentice-Hall, 1980. ISBN: 0139619461.

Kaufman, Miriam, M.D. and Teresa Pitman: *All Shapes and Sizes*. Canada: HarperCollins, 1994. ISBN: 0-00-638020-4.

Kaz-Cooke: *Real Gorgeous*. W W Norton & Company, 1996. ISBN: 0393313557.

Klein, Richard: *Eat Fat*. New York: Pantheon Books, 1996. ISBN: 0679441972.

Kratina, Karin, M.A., R.D., L.D.; Nancy L. King, M.S., R.D., C.D.E.; and Dayle Hayes, M.S., R.D., L.D: ***Moving Away From Diets***. Helm Seminars, Publishing, 1996.

Lamb, Wally: *She's Come Undone*. New York: Washington Square Press, 1996. ISBN: 0671003755.

Langer, Stephen with James F. Scheer: Solved: *The Riddle of Weight Loss*. Rochester, VT: Healing Arts Press, 1989. ISBN: 0892812966.

Lewis, Mark. with a foreword by Les Dawson: *The Roly Polys : fit, fat and fruity*. London: W.H. Allen, 1986. ISBN: 0491031750.

Lidell, Lucy: *The Sensual Body*. New York: Simon and Schuster, Inc., A Fireside Book, 1987. ISBN: 0671660330.

Lippincott, Catherine: *Well Rounded: Eight Simple Steps for Changing Your Life...Not Your Size.* New York: Pocket Books, 1997. ISBN: 0671545086.

Lyons, Pat and Debby Burgard: *Great Shape: The First Fitness Guide for Large Women.* iUniverse.com, Inc., 2000. ISBN: 059508883X.

Mackoff, Barbara Dr.: *Growing A Girl : Seven Strategies For Raising A Strong Spirited Daughter.* New York: Dell Publishing, 1996. ISBN: 0440506611.

Mann, Dr. George. "The Influence of Obesity on Health." *New England Journal of Medicine,* July-August 1974.

Marano, Hara Estroff: *Style is Not a Size.* New York: Bantam Books, 1991. ISBN: 0553352709.

Mayer, Ken: *Real Women Don't Diet!.* Silver Spring, MD: Bartleby Press, 1993. ISBN: 0910155275.

Millman, Marcia: *Such a Pretty Face: Being Fat in America.* New York: Norton, 1980. ISBN: 0393013170.

Milne, A.A: *The World of Christopher Robin.* New York: E P Dutton, 1958 / Reissue edition 1988. ISBN: 0525444483.

Murray, Lynne: *Larger Than Death.* Athens, GA: Orloff Press, 1997. ISBN: 0-9642949-0-7.

Naidus, Beverly: *One Size Does Not Fit All.* Littleton: Aigis Publications, 1993. ISBN: 1883930006.

Nanfeldt, Suzan: *Plus Style: The Plus-Size Guide to Looking Great.* New York: Dutton, 1996. ISBN: 0-452-27596-2.

Newman, Leslea and Michael Willhoite: *Belinda's Bouquet.* Boston: Alyson Wonderland Publications, 1991. ISBN: 1-55583-154-0.

Newman, Leslea, ed: *Eating Our Hearts Out: Personal Accounts of Women's Relationship to Food.* Freedom, CA: The Crossing Press, 1993. ISBN: 0-89594-569-X.

Newman, Leslea: *Fat Chance*. New York: G.P. Putnam Sons, 1994. ISBN: 0-39-922760-1.

Newman, Leslea: *Some Body to Love*. Chicago: Third Side Press, 1992. ISBN: 1-879427-03-6.

Northrup, Christiane, M.D: *Women's Bodies, Women's Wisdom: Creating Physical and Emotional Health and Healing*. New York: Bantam Books, 1994. ISBN: 0553081209.

Notkin, Debbie and Laurie Toby Edison: *Women En Large: Images of Fat Nudes*. City: Books in Focus, 1994. ISBN: 1-885495-00-5.

Odean, Kathleen: *Great Books for Girls: More Than 600 Books To Inspire Today's Girls And Tomorrow's Women*. New York: Ballantine Books, 1997. ISBN: 034540484X.

O'Gaden, Irene: *Fat Girl: One Woman's Way Out*. San Francisco: Harper San Francisco, 1993. ISBN: 0-06-250727-3.

Ogden, Jane: *Fat Chance! The Myth of Dieting Explained*. London and New York: Routledge, 1992. ISBN: 0415073715.

Olds, Ruthanne: *Big and Beautiful : Become the Big Beautiful Person You Were Meant to Be*. Washington: Acropolis Books, 1982. ISBN: 0874910889.

Omichinski, Linda R.D: ***You Count, Calories Don't.*** Hyperion Press, Canada, 1992.

Orbach, Susie: *Fat Is a Feminist Issue II: A Program to Conquer Compulsive Eating*. New York: Berkley Books, 1982. ISBN: 0425056422.

Orbach, Susie: *Fat Is a Feminist Issue*. New York: Berkley Publishing Corporation, A Berkley Book, 1978. ISBN: 0425040356.

Orenstein, Peggy: *School Girls - **Young Women, Self-Esteem, and the Confidence Gap***. New York: Doubleday, 1994. ISBN: 0385425759.

Pinkwater, Daniel: *The Afterlife Diet*. New York: Random House, 1995. ISBN: 0679419365.

Pipher, Mary: *Hunger Pains : The Modern Woman's Tragic Quest for Thinness*. New York: Ballantine Books, 1997. ISBN: 0345413938.

Pipher, Mary: *Reviving Ophelia : **Saving the Selves of Adolescent Girls***. New York: Ballantine Books, 1995. ISBN: 0345392825.

Poulton, Terry. *No Fat Chicks: How Big Business Profits Making Women Hate Their Bodies-How to Fight Back*. Secaucus: Carol Publishing Group, A Birch Lane Press Book, 1997. ISBN: 1559724234.

Roberts, Nancy: *Breaking All the Rules*. New York: Viking Penguin, Inc., 1987. ISBN: 0140074635.

Rodin, Judith: *Body Traps: Breaking the Binds that Keep You from Feeling Good About Your Body*. New York: William Morrow and Company, Inc., 1992. ISBN: 0688088430.

Rose, Laura: *Life Isn't Weighed on the Bathroom Scales; Don't Be a Victim of the Thinness Conspiracy*. WRS Group, Inc., 1994. ISBN: 1567960375.

Roth, Geneen: *Breaking Free from Compulsive Eating*. Indianapolis: Bobbs-Merrill, 1984. ISBN: 067252810X.

Roth, Geneen: *Feeding the Hungry Heart: The Experience of Compulsive Eating*. Indianapolis: Bobbs-Merrill, 1982. ISBN: 0672527316.

Rush, Anne Kent: *Getting Clear: Body Work for Women*. New York: Random House, 1973.

Sabo, Sandie: *Sandie's Clothesline*. $15.95 to Sandie Sabo, PO Box 257, Cardiff by the Sea, CA 92007.

Sabo, Sandie: *So you want to be a model!.* $14.95 to Sandie Sabo, PO Box 257, Cardiff by the Sea, CA 92007.

Schroeder, Charles Roy: *Fat Is Not a Four-Letter Word.* Minneapolis: Chronimed Publishing, 1992. ISBN: 1-56561-000-8.

Schwartz, Bob: *Diets Don't Work.* Breakthru Publishing, 1996. ISBN: 0942540166.

Schwartz, Hillel: *Never Satisfied: A Cultural History of Diets, Fantasies, and Fat.* New York: The Free Press / London: Collier Macmillan, 1986. ISBN: 0029292506.

Seid, Roberta Pollack: *Never Too Thin: Why Women Are at War with Their Bodies.* New York: Prentice Hall Press, 1989. ISBN: 0139251162.

Seligman, Martin E. P: *What You Can Change...And What You Can't: The Complete Guide to Successful Self-Improvement and Learning to Accept Who You Are.* New York: Knopf, 1994. ISBN: 0679410244.

Shaw, Carole and Hank Nuwer: *Come Out, Come Out, Wherever You Are.* Los Angeles: American R. R. Publishing Company, 1982.

Siegel, Michele, Judith Brisman & Margot Weinshel: *Surviving An Eating Disorder : New Perspectives and Strategies for Family and Friends.* New York: Harper & Row, 1988. ISBN: 0060915536.

Solovay, Sondra: *Tipping the Scales of Justice: Fighting Weight Based Discrimination.* Amherst: Prometheus Books, 2000. ISBN: 1-57392-764-3.

Sommers, Abigail: *Love in the Pyramid.* Rubenesque Romances, PO Box 534, Tarrytown, NY 10591-0534. (800) 211-1660. ISBN: 1-888038-04-7

St. Paige, Edward: *Zaftig: The Case for Curves.* Blue Lantern Books, 1999. ISBN: 1883211174.

Stacey, Michelle: *Consumed: Why Americans Love, Hate, and Fear Food.* New York: Simon & Schuster, 1994. ISBN: 0671767542.

Stimson, Karen: *Fat Feminist Herstory.* Largesse Presse, PO Box 9404, New Haven, CT 06534.

Stimson, Karen: *Room To Grow.* Largesse Presse, PO Box 9404, New Haven, CT 06534.

Stinson, Susan: *Belly Songs: In celebration of fat women.* PO Box 433, Northhampton, MA 01060.

Stinson, Susan: *Fat Girl Dances with Rocks.* Minneapolis: Spinsters Ink, 1994. ISBN: 1883523028.

Stinson, Susan: **Martha Moody.** Duluth: Spinsters Ink, 1995. ISBN: 1883523079.

Straw, William E: *Stop Dieting Before It Kills You.* PRC Publishing, 1997. ISBN: 0944183212.

Stuart, Mary S. and Lynnzy Orr: *Otherwise Perfect: People and Their Problems with Weight.* Pompano Beach, FL: Health Communications, Inc., 1987. ISBN: 0932194575.

Stuart, Richard B. and Barbara Jacobson: *Weight, Sex & Marriage: A Delicate Balance.* New York: Simon & Schuster, A Fireside Book, 1989. ISBN: 0671670085.

Stunkard, Albert J., M.D: *The Pain of Obesity.* Palo Alto: Bull Publishing Co., 1976. ISBN: 0915950057.

Sullivan, Judy: *Size Wise.* New York: Avon Books, 1997.

Sward, Sharon: *You Are More Than What You Weigh: Improving Your Self Esteem No Matter What Your Weight.* Wholesome Publisher, 1995. ISBN: 0-96488-740-1.

Thompson, Becky W: *A Hunger So Wide and So Deep.* Minneapolis: University of Minnesota Press, 1994. ISBN: 0816624348.

Thone, Ruth: *Fat--A Fate Worse Than Death? Women, Weight, and Appearance.* New York: Haworth Press, 1997. ISBN: 1560239085.

Toronto INDD Coalition: **Foxy Fables and Facts About Dieting: A Journey to Healthy Lifestyles.** NEDIC, Canada, 1996.

Walker, Elizabeth Neff: *An Abundant Woman.* Belgrave House, 1998. ISBN: 0966064372.

Wann, Marilyn: *FAT!SO? Because You Don't Have to Apologize for Your Size.* Berkeley: Ten Speed Press, 1998. ISBN: 0898159954.

Wiley, Carol, ed: *Journeys to Self-Acceptance: Fat Women Speak.* Freedom, CA: The Crossing Press, 1994. ISBN: 0-89594-656-4.

Wolf, Naomi: *The Beauty Myth: How Images of Beauty Are Used Against Women.* New York: William Morrow & Co., 1991. ISBN: 0688510508.

Yetiv, Jack Z: *Popular Nutritional Practices: Sense and Nonsense.* New York: Dell, 1988.

Young, Mary Evans: **Diet Breaking: Having it All Without Having to Diet.** UK: Hodder & Stoughton, 1995. ISBN: 0340637900.

References

Introduction

Clinical Guidelines on the Identification, Evaluation, and Treatment of Overweight and Obesity in Adults – The Evidence Report. Bethesda, Md: National Heart, Lung, and Blood Institute; reprint June 1998:

Van Horn L, Donato K, Kumanyika S, Wonston M, Prewitt E, and Snetselaar L. The dietitian's role in the developing and implementing the first federal obesity guidelines. *J Am Diet Assoc*. 1998;98:1115-1117

Kassirer JP, Angell M. Losing weight—an ill-fated new year's resolution [editorial]. *N Engl J Med*. 1998;338:52-54

Polivy J. Psychological consequences of food restriction. *J Am Diet Assoc*. 1996;96:589-592

Wooley SC, Garner DM. Obesity treatment: the high cost of false hope. *J Am Diet Assoc*. 1991;91:1248-1251.

Manore MM. Chronic dieting in active women: what are the health consequences? *Women's Health Issues*. 1996;6:332-341.

Van Loan M. Ikeda JP. Restrained eating and bone density in women. *Healthscene West.* 1997;11:1-4.

Chapter 1: A New Way of Thinking

Bennett, William and Joel Gurin: *The Dieter's Dilemma: Eating Less and Weighing More.* New York: Basic Books, 1982; 38-47.

Neumark-Sztainer D, Butler R, Palti H. Personal and socioenvironmental predictors of disordered eating among adolescent females. J Nutr Educ. 1996;28:195-201.

Hill AJ, Draper J, Stack M. A weight on children's minds: Body shape dissatisfaction at 9 years old. Int J Obes Relat Metab Disord. 1994;18:383-389

Hirschmann, Jane R. and Carol H. Munter: *Overcoming Overeating.* Reading, MA: Addison-Wesley Publishing Company, Inc., 1988; 212-230

Wilfley DE, Schreiber GB, Pike KM, Streigel-Moore RH, Wright DJ, Rodin J. Eating disturbances and body image: a comparison of a community sample of adult black and white women. *Int J Eating Disord.* 1996;20:377-387.

Rolland K, Farnill D, Griffiths RA. Body figure perception and eating attitudes among Australilan Schoolchildren age 8 to 12 years. *Int J Obes.* 1997;21:273-278

Weight war worsening. *Sough China Morning Post,* June 10, 1998.

Robinson JI, HoerrSL, Petersmarck KA, Anderson JV, Redefining success on obesity intervention: the new paradigm. *J Am Diet Assoc*. 1995;95:422-423

Hayes DM. Body Trust—undieting your way to health and happiness. *Radiance*—the Magazine for Large Women. 1995;12:42-46

OgdenJ, Evans C. The problem with weighing: effects on mood, self-esteem, and body image. *Int J Obes Relat Metab Disord*. 1996;20:272-277.

Wooley, O. W., S. W. Wooley, and S. R. Dyrenforth. "Obesity and Women--I. A Closer Look at the Facts" and "Obesity and Women--II. A Neglected Feminist Topic." *Women's Studies International Quarterly*, 2 (1979), 69-79, 81-92.

Chapter 2: Making Peace with Food

Garner DMm Wooley SC, Confronting the failure of behavioral and dietary treatments for obesity. *Clin Psychol Rev*. 1991;11:729-780

Leibel RL, Rosenbaum M, hirsch J. Changes in energy expinditure resulting from altered body weight. *N Engl M J Med*. 1995;332:621-628.

Schwartz MW, Seeley RJ. The new Biology of body weight regulation. *J Am Diet Assoc*. 1997;97:54-58

Wickelgren I. Obesity: how big a problem? *Science*. 1998;280:1364-1367

Lynn, Thom N. et al. "Prevalence of Evidence of Prior Myocardial Infarction, Hypertension, and Diabetes with Obesity in Three Neighboring Communities in Pennsylvania." *The American Journal of the Medical Sciences*, October 1967, 385-391.

Appel J, Moore TJ, Obarzanek E, Bollmer WM, Svetsky LP, Sacks FM, Bray GA, Bogt TM, Cutler JA, Windhauser MM, Lin PH, Karanja N. A clinical trial of the effects of dietary patterns on blood pressure. *N Eng J Med.* 1997;336:1117-1124

Chapter 3: Fitness and Motivation

Bennett, William and Joel Gurin: *The Dieter's Dilemma: Eating Less and Weighing More.* New York: Basic Books, 1982; 100-106.

Barlow CE, Khol HW III, Gibbons LW, Blair SN. Physical fitness, mortality, and obesity. *Int J Obes.* 1995;19(suppl4):S41-S44.

Fraser, Laura: *Losing It: America's Obsession With Weight and the Industry That Feeds on It.* New York: Dutton, 1997; 268-276.

Narayan KM, Hoskin M, Kazak D, Kriska AM, Hanson RL, Pettitt DJ, Natgi DK, Bennet PH, Knowler WC. Randomized clinical trial of lifestylke interventions in Pima Indians: a pilot study. *Diabetic Med.* 1998;15:66-72.

Gaesser, Glenn A: *Big Fat Lies: The Truth About Your Weight and Your Health.* New York: Fawcett Columbine, 1996; 205-211, 224-227.

Lynch J, Helmrich SP, Lakka TA, Kaplan GA, Cohen RD, Salonen R, Salonen JT, Moderately intense physical activities and high levels of cardiorespiratory fitness reduce risk of non-insulin-dependent diabetes mellitus in middle aged men. *Arch Intern Med.* 1996;156:1307-1314

Lyons, Pat and Debby Burgard: *Great Shape: The First Fitness Guide for Large Women.* iUniverse.com, Inc., 2000; 156-160.

Barnard RJ, Effects of lifestyle modifications on serum lipids, *Arch Intern Med.* 1991;151:1389-1394

Brown MD, Moore GE, Korytowski MT, McCole SE, Habberg JM. Improvement of insulin sensitivity by short-term exercise training in hypertensive African-American women. *Hypertension.* 1997;30:1549-1553.

Stout, Clark et al. "Unusually Low Incidence of Death from Myocardial Infarction." *Journal of the American Medical Association*, v. 188, n. 10, 845-849.

Lemaitre R, et al. *Arch Intern Med.* 1999;159:686-690

Chapter 4: Putting It All Together

Dulloo AG, Jacquet J, Gorardier L. Post starvation hyperphagia and body fat overshooting. *Am J Clin Nutr.* 1997;65:717-723

Stice E, Cameron RP, Hayward C, et al. Naturalistic weight reduction efforts prospectively predict growth in relative weight and onset of obesity among female adolescents. *J Consuld Clin Psychol.* 1999;67:967-974

Lee Im, Paffenbarger RS Jr. Is weight loss hazardous? Increased mortality for those who cycled in their weight found in 5 different studies. *Nutr Rev.* 1996;54 (suppl):S116-S124.

Kassirer JP, Angell M. Losing weight—an ill-fated new year's resolution [editorial]. *N Engl J Med.* 1998;338:52-54

Polivy J. Psychological consequences of food restriction. *J Am Diet Assoc.* 1996;96:589-592

Wooley SC, Garner DM. Obesity treatment: the high cost of false hope. *J Am Diet Assoc.* 1991;91:1248-1251.

Index

Order Your Fitness Videos by Kelly Bliss

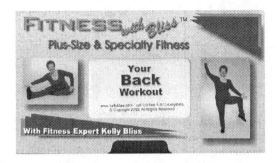

Order online at www.kellybliss.com
Call toll free 877-KellyBliss (877-535-5925)

Only $19.95 per video (plus $8 s&h)

Get 15% off! Order three or more videos
Only 16.95 per video (plus $10 s&h total)

Mail Your Order:

Name _____

Address _____

City _____ State _____ Zip _____

(Please make checks payable to Work It Out, Inc.)

Charge: _____ Visa _____ MC _____ AMEX _____ Discover

Acct # _____

Exp date: _____ Amt: _____

Mail your order to P.O. Box 572, Lansdowne, PA 19050-1406

Video Name _____

Video Name _____

Video Name _____

Video Name _____

1. The FORM workout

This is a lower intensity workout with lots of information about correct form and posture.

2. No-impact Aerobics II

This standing aerobics workout is medium intensity. If you can walk a few blocks comfortably, then you can do this workout.

3. No-impact Aerobics III

This faster paced workout is higher intensity, yet still has NO jumping. If you can power walk (or walk fast) for several blocks, then you can do this workout.

4. Sitting Aerobics I

Do you have trouble standing or walking for any reason? Then grab a chair and get ready to boogie!

5. Sitting Aerobics II

Do you need to workout sitting down, but also you want a more intense aerobic workout? Then this is the workout for you! (Note: If you are a person who uses a wheelchair, you can follow along with any sitting workout and do the movements that work for you and your body.)

6. Muscle Toning I

Do you get a pain in the neck just thinking about "crunches"? In this workout you can work your abdominal muscles sitting up! Nice lower intensity exercises for abs, buns, legs, back, and arms.

7. Muscle Toning II

This muscle-toning workout can also be done on the comfortable surface of your bed or on an exercise mat on the floor. Every step of the way, you will learn how to strengthen and protect your muscles and joints.

8. Your Back Health Workout

This workout is also great for people who cope with chronic pain. In this workout, you will enjoy smooth moves standing, sitting, and reclining. CHECK WITH YOUR DOCTOR. If you have back pain from skeletal or disc problems, this may or may not be appropriate for you - CHECK WITH YOUR DOCTOR.

9. Stretch and Relax for small to large people:
Enjoy gentle warm-up moves and stretches that you WILL be able to do. These moves are appropriate for small people and for large people. (Note: if you are a very large person, over 300#, check out Stretch and Relax for very large people)

10. Stretch and Relax for very large people:
In this work out you will enjoy stretches and movements that you CAN do. There is room for all of you here! You can work on a bed or a large couch where you can recline and stretch.

Kelly still provides "Self-Care Coaching" by phone!

Yes, Kelly is committed to continuing her work with individuals. She offers her services at very affordable rates. You are welcome to give her a call and see if there is an opening in her schedule for you to become one of her clients. 610-394-2547

If you live in the Philadelphia area check www.KellyBliss.com for the "Philly Classes" or call toll free for a schedule.

Fitness with Bliss Exercise Classes

Healthy Eating with Bliss Groups

1-877-KellyBliss
1-877-535-5925